SURVEY SCALES

Also Available

*Assessing Performance:
Designing, Scoring, and Validating
Performance Tasks*
Robert L. Johnson, James A. Penny,
and Belita Gordon

SURVEY SCALES

A Guide to Development, Analysis, and Reporting

ROBERT L. JOHNSON
GRANT B. MORGAN

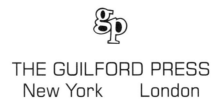

THE GUILFORD PRESS
New York   London

© 2016 The Guilford Press
A Division of Guilford Publications, Inc.
370 Seventh Avenue, Suite 1200, New York, NY 10001
www.guilford.com

Printed in the United States of America

This book is printed on acid-free paper.

Last digit is print number: 9   8   7   6   5   4   3   2   1

Library of Congress Cataloging-in-Publication Data is available
from the publisher.

ISBN 978-1-4625-2696-3 (paperback)
ISBN 978-1-4625-2697-0 (hardcover)

To our families

Mildred and Walter, my parents
Judy, Jerri, and Jeannie, my sisters
Richard, my partner
—R. L. J.

Olivia, my daughter
Jessica, my wife
Cheryl, my mom
—G. B. M.

Preface

When you opened this book, you probably were looking for the answers to some questions, such as:

- "When I am writing items, how do I ensure the items are targeting the focus of my research?"
- "If I use a few items from another researcher's scale, do I need to obtain copyright permission to use the items?"
- "How do I decide which items are 'good' and which are 'problematic'?"
- "Should the scales on the items be 4-point, 5-point, or more?"
- "Should each scale point have a label?"
- "How do I investigate the reliability and validity associated with the survey scale?"

We wrote *Survey Scales: A Guide to Development, Analysis, and Reporting* to answer these questions (and some others). We also wrote it to provide a resource for those in research and program evaluation who plan to develop scales for use in surveys by explaining such topics as:

- Reviewing existing scales for use in a study,
- Designing a framework to guide scale development,
- Writing items,

- Developing item response scales,
- Examining validity and reliability,
- Conducting a factor analysis,
- Analyzing data, and
- Reporting scale results.

In *Survey Scales*, we synthesize the literature from the survey and measurement fields. The book is grounded in our research and experience in conducting surveys, as well as feedback from our students in the survey design courses we've taught. Since the literature on scale development is not always consistent in its guidance on design, *Survey Scales* is written to help readers select the appropriate methodology or approach to use and understand why such methods or approaches are appropriate. Rather than focus on a single discipline, we draw examples from various professional fields, such as education, psychology, and public health.

Survey Scales is applied in that it is a resource for those who plan to use survey scales in a research study or an evaluation. It will be of interest to practitioners who are planning a survey as well as to doctoral students who are developing surveys to use in data collection for their dissertations. We begin at the first step in scale development and end with analyzing data and reporting results, so it may be helpful for first-time readers to take the chapters in sequence. We purposely ordered the chapters in such a way that scale developers will have food for thought and guidance for each step of the development process.

Researchers may find the coverage of frameworks for scale development (Chapter 3) particularly useful because this is an area that is not commonly addressed in other texts. We have carefully presented the information so that readers can follow and begin creating their own frameworks for scale development. Having such a framework is an excellent way to identify the critical components of an instrument and ensure that desired elements are included in the scale.

For those readers who may have an existing instrument in mind, we have also included a chapter on adopting or adapting existing scales (Chapter 2). In this chapter, we present criteria for determining whether a preexisting scale is likely to provide data of an appropriate quality for a research study or program evaluation. Readers are introduced to the *Mental Measurements Yearbook*, a resource that provides critiques of measurement tools, such as attitude scales. Chapter 2 also provides guidance on the use of journal articles to find information about the technical quality of scales. In addition, we provide guidance on the extent to which a researcher can appropriately incorporate items or sections of a survey scale into his or her scale and on the need to obtain permission to use copyrighted scales.

For readers who will be writing items for their own research or evaluations, our chapter on item-writing guidelines (Chapter 4) will be especially useful. In Chapter 4, we introduce strategies that will help survey developers to write items that are clear to the respondents and assess the construct of interest. Throughout the chapter we provide a range of examples. In these examples, we use a "Not This/But This" feature to present problematic items (i.e., "NOT THIS") and specific strategies for revising the items (i.e., "BUT THIS").

The chapter on rating scale development (Chapter 5) specifically discusses considerations for the number of appropriate levels for an item response scale, the use of odd or even number of levels, verbal labels and descriptors, and the directionality of statements and response scales. The formatting and piloting chapter (Chapter 6) discusses formatting items and specific stakeholders who may review items prior to administration.

With regard to analyzing data collected using survey scales, we have provided three chapters that are written in a very accessible, reader-friendly manner. We begin with a discussion of descriptive statistics (Chapter 7), which includes examples of many types of analyses. In Chapter 8, we present the concepts of validity and reliability. The chapter describes methods for collecting evidence about the degree to which the survey scale is likely to contribute to valid decisions based on the data from the scale. In Chapter 9, we introduce and demonstrate the use of exploratory factor analysis. Factor analysis is used to examine whether a survey scale is unidimensional, in which case a single scale score is appropriate, or multidimensional, in which case reporting multiple subscale scores might be appropriate.

Another topic that is commonly overlooked in other texts is reporting the results of survey scales through the use of tables and graphs. In Chapter 10, we provide specific guidance about the construction of tables and graphs to summarize data from surveys. We also discuss the use of tables and graphs to show the relationship(s) between results from a survey scale and other variables.

In *Survey Scales*, readers will find suggestions for further readings, exercises with sample answers from the authors, a glossary of key terms, and an appendix that reviews basic principles of inferential statistics as well as examples of parametric and nonparametric procedures that may be useful for group comparisons.

We would like to thank Jordan Litman, Department of Psychology, University of North Florida, along with other anonymous reveiwers, for their constructive comments and insights, which resulted in a more useful final product. We would also like to thank our editor at The Guilford Press, C. Deborah Laughton, for her guidance and patience in this process. We extend our thanks to Xuegang Zhang for his feedback on the item-writing chapters. We also want to express our appreciation to Diane Monradin in the South Carolina Educational Center, Tammiee Dickenson in the Office of Program Evaluation, and Jeff Potts in the Office of Assessment and Accountability in Richland School District Two. We hope that the implementation and documentation of the strategies described in *Survey Scales* will assist readers in developing survey scales that support accurate decisions in research and program evaluation. We hope that you, the reader, enjoy learning from this text, and we welcome feedback from you about new topics or methodologies that we should incorporate in future editions of *Survey Scales*.

Brief Contents

Extended Contents

9. Factor Analysis   143

10. Documenting the Development of the Survey Scale   171

Scales in Surveys

*To conduct research is to collect, analyze, and interpret **data** systematically so as to answer specific questions about a **phenomenon** of interest.*
—CHOW (2010, p. 1260)

Introduction

Chow's quote highlights the role of data in conducting **survey** research. Data collection helps us to answer questions about a phenomenon of interest (i.e., an activity, process, or program that is the research focus). Data collection in a research study helps us to investigate client satisfaction with a service, student attitudes toward school, consumer buying behaviors, and public knowledge of the benefits of nutritional supplements. Data can take the form of responses to survey items, ratings from observations, and scores on knowledge-based tests.

Examples of the types of data provided by surveys include customer responses to satisfaction scales when purchasing a car. During elections, the responses of survey participants provide information about likely voters' preferences for president. At the university level, students complete course evaluations at the end of the semester to provide feedback about their professors. Program evaluations use surveys to solicit feedback about the services provided by a project. To develop licensure examinations that will determine whether a recent graduate in nursing will be allowed to practice, experts in the field of nursing respond to survey items to indicate job tasks that are critical in the execution of their professional responsibilities.

Surveys include closed-response and **open-response items** (see Figure 1.1). Open-response items require a survey participant to form his or her answer. In contrast, **closed-response items** provide answer options from

1

Example of a Closed-Response Survey Item				
Academic skills and preparation	Strongly disagree	Disagree	Agree	Strongly agree
I received the help I needed to improve my academic skills this year.	1	2	3	4

Example of an Open-Response Survey Item
As a senior, what advice would you give eighth graders that would make their move into ninth grade easier?

FIGURE 1.1. Example of a closed- and an open-response survey item.

which the survey participant selects a response. As shown in Table 1.1, each format has its advantages and disadvantages.

Closed-Response Items

Advantages of closed-response items include assuring that the survey respondents consider issues important to the study. If, for example, you ask an open-response question about the strengths and weakness of respondents' recent visit to their health care provider, the survey participants might not address the quality of services provided by the nurses and medical assistants. Closed-response items focus participants' attention on the issues presented in the answer options. If all respondents consider the same issues, then the data can be used in statistical comparisons across groups. Another advantage of closed-response items is their appeal to survey participants who are reluctant to respond to items that require lengthy written responses. In addition, responses to these items can be reliably entered into a database for analysis.

Disadvantages of closed-response items include the need for the researcher to know all relevant answer options for an item. Thus, potential answer options must be generated during the development of the instrument. Another disadvantage is the fact that the study findings are in the language of the researcher. That is, the researcher's conceptualization frames the study findings, and the views of the study participants might not be expressed.

Open-Response Items

An advantage of open-response items is the potential to gain unanticipated responses from survey participants. In addition, the open-response format provides respondents with an opportunity to express their views and allows

TABLE 1.1. Closed- and Open-Response Items

Type	Characteristics	Advantages	Disadvantages
Closed-response items	Items composed of a stem and answer options. Respondent selects from predetermined options.	Ensures coverage of issues important to the researcher. Focuses respondents' attention on the issues that are presented in a set of answer options. Useful for those reluctant to provide lengthy written responses. Provides uniform data across groups and allows statistical comparison of those groups. Reliable data entry and analysis.	Must know answer options prior to the construction of the survey. Findings framed in the language of the researcher and might not express the views of the survey participants.
Open-response items	A statement or question to which a survey participant responds. For written responses, an item typically includes a blank or box to record the respondent's answers. In an interview, the survey participant's response is taped or recorded in written field notes.	Gain unanticipated answers. Research findings in the language of the survey participants and can include quotes. Provides respondents with an opportunity to express their views. Useful when surveying about a topic about which little is known.	Respondent might not consider all aspects of the phenomenon being studied. Requires more time to administer the survey, enter responses into a database, and analyze the information, so less breadth in issues covered and fewer respondents. Demands of writing responses might lose those with literacy challenges. Respondents tend to skip open-response items. Requires development of a coding system. Consistency of coding presents challenges.

Note. Summarized from Dillman, Smyth, and Christian (2009); Fink (2013); and Fowler (2014).

the researcher to use quotes to express study findings in the language of the survey participants. Responses to open-response items also can be used to generate answer options for use in closed-response items in future studies.

Disadvantages of open-response items include a tendency for respondents to skip this type of item. Also, respondents do not focus on the same aspects of a research phenomenon; thus statistical comparisons across groups are not possible. Verbal answers to open-response items require time and financial resources for coding. Also, the consistency of the coding can be a challenge. After data are coded, the analysis takes a substantial amount of time. With these demands on time and resources, an investigator might be faced with limiting the study to fewer survey participants and narrowing the scope of the study.

In order to capture the benefit of open- and closed-response items, researchers frequently include a mix of item types in a survey. At other times, the research focus leads survey developers to develop a collection of closed-response items to measure respondents' attitudes, behaviors, or knowledge. Such a collection of items is often referred to as a scale and is used to measure **constructs** (i.e., abstract concepts), such as attitudes, along a continuum. In addition, a survey might contain multiple scales, such as a high school survey with two different scales related to Student Engagement and School Climate.

The focus of *Survey Scales: A Guide to Development, Analysis, and Reporting* is on the development of closed-response items. We consider the use of checklists, true–false variations, and Likert-style items (see Figure

Checklists	3. I have participated in the following this past year. (Check **ALL** that apply.) ____ Tutoring and Testing Center ____ Freshman seminars ____ Freshman Mentoring Program[1]
True–false variations	9. If you are a vegetarian, you probably will need to take a supplement for vitamins D and B12 as you age. A. True B. False[2]
Likert-style items	To provide us with information about your experience at the clinic please rate the following: 1. The doctor taking time to answer your questions 1 Very poor 2 Poor 3 Good 4 Very good

FIGURE 1.2. Examples of closed-response survey items. [1]Johnson, Monrad, Amsterdam, and May (2005); [2]University of Arkansas for Medical Sciences (2014).

1.2). Checklists serve as one method to measure behaviors and knowledge. True–false variations also are useful in measuring survey respondents' knowledge. Likert-style items are the dominant method used to measure attitudes (Riconscente & Romeo, 2010; Scholderer, 2011).

An Overview of the Survey Scale Development Process

In this section, we provide an overview of the process of developing a **survey scale**. Figure 1.3 lists the major steps in the construction of a survey scale.

Establish the Purpose of a Survey

As shown in Figure 1.3, a critical first step in developing a survey scale is to identify the purpose of the research study. Is the purpose of the survey to collect data to investigate a research question? For example, a survey could ask teachers about their assessment practices to investigate the following research question:

Identify the purpose of a survey.

- Investigate a research question.
- Conduct a needs assessment.
- Evaluate a program.
- Inform accountability.

Define the constructs and their relationships.

- Conduct a literature review.
- Develop a conceptual framework.

Review potential scales for adoption or adaptation.

Write items and response scales.

Format the survey.

- Determine administration method (e.g., web, interview).

Submit the instrument for review.

- Submit for content, editorial, and bias reviews.
- Pilot the survey.

Field test the survey and analyze data to make final changes.

Document the development of the survey scale.

FIGURE 1.3. The survey development process.

How are teachers' uses of various types of classroom assessments,
such as multiple-choice items, paper- and pencil-based writing, and
oral communication, related to their fourth graders' achievement in
reading for literary experience and reading for acquiring and using
information?
(Hao & Johnson, 2013)

Will the survey assist in the conduct of a needs assessment? The purpose of such a survey might be to determine the needs of arts educators as
they prepare to assume the role of evaluators and conduct evaluations of
arts programs. Answers to such a survey would inform the development
of a graduate course that would address the needs of the future program
evaluators in the visual and performing arts.

Is the purpose of the survey to collect data to evaluate programs? Surveys could inform such evaluation questions as "To what extent do teachers' lesson plans reflect the incorporation of visual and performing arts
standards into instruction?" and "What is the quality of staff development
opportunities being offered?"

Some surveys are used to meet state and national accountability reg-
ulations. An example is South Carolina's accountability legislation that
requires the inclusion of climate data in school, district, and state report
cards (Monrad et al., 2008). School climate data are collected by surveying
parents, teachers, and students. To collect information from these groups,
South Carolina annually administers school climate surveys. Examples of
items on *The South Carolina Teacher Survey* include "The school leadership makes a sustained effort to address teacher concerns." and "I feel supported by administrators at my school" (Monrad et al., 2008).

Define the Construct

After identifying the purpose of the survey, the next step is to define the
constructs that constitute the phenomenon of interest. A construct is an
abstract instance of a **concept**. That is, a construct is an attribute or idea—
a concept—that is not directly observable (Hopkins, 1998). Constructs are
the structures or processes that are theorized to underlie observed phenomena (Gall, Gall, & Borg, 2010). A construct might be composed of multiple
domains. These domains are also referred to as **components**.

An example of a construct and its domains is "student engagement."
Shown in Figure 1.4 is a survey scale with items that ask about students'
participating in class and their getting along with others. Are the items in
Figure 1.4 measuring two different domains—academic engagement and
social engagement—that constitute the student engagement construct? One
way to answer this question is to review the literature and researchers'

Participating in Class—Academic Engagement				
6. As a ninth-grade student **I . . .**	**Rarely**	**Sometimes**	**Often**	**All the time**
a. enjoy learning new things.	1	2	3	4
b. complete all my work.	1	2	3	4
c. need more help to understand the classwork.	1	2	3	4
d. come to class without books, pencil, or paper.	1	2	3	4
e. read the materials that are being talked about in class.	1	2	3	4
f. make notes about what I read.	1	2	3	4
g. study to prepare for tests.		2	3	4
h. skip classes.	1	2	3	4
Getting Along with Others—Social Engagement				
7. As a ninth-grade student **I . . .**	**Strongly disagree**	**Disagree**	**Agree**	**Strongly agree**
a. have many friends at school.	1	2	3	4
b. care if I finish high school.	1	2	3	4
c. care what other students think about me.	1	2	3	4
d. care what teachers think about me.	1	2	3	4
e. know what my teachers expect of me.	1	2	3	4
f. talk with adults (teachers, counselors, coaches) when I have problems.	1	2	3	4
g. often get sent to an administrator for misbehaving.	1	2	3	4

FIGURE 1.4. Examples of types of closed-response items that measure domains related to student engagement. Adapted from Johnson, Davis, Fisher, Johnson, and Somerindyke (2000). Copyright © 2000 Richland School District Two, Columbia, South Carolina. Adapted by permission.

conceptualization of "student engagement." If the construct is considered to encompass the domains of both academic and social engagement, then construction of your survey will involve operationalizing the construct domains by writing items to develop two **subscales** similar to those in Figure 1.4. That is, items in the subscales will serve as individual **indicators** of the underlying construct and **operationalize** the abstract construct of student engagement into two **variables** (i.e., academic engagement and social engagement).

Variables refer to characteristics that take on different values for different study participants. For example, on a survey of student engagement, some participants will respond favorably (e.g., "Strongly agree") to statements related to academic engagement, whereas other students will respond less positively (e.g., "Strongly disagree"). Thus, scores on the academic engagement scale vary across students. Unlike abstract, unobservable constructs, variables can be used to investigate a phenomenon of interest, such as whether the student engagement variables predict successful student transition (i.e., promotion) from ninth to tenth grade.

Listed in Table 1.2 are examples of survey scales that measure an array of constructs. In the conduct of a study, researchers and evaluators measure such constructs as attitudes toward diversity, job satisfaction, student engagement, and perceptions about the ethics of classroom assessment practices. Note that some of these constructs are composed of multiple domains or subscales, such as the Caregiver Survey, which comprises the domains of job satisfaction, supervisory relationships, and job environment. Other constructs are composed of only one domain, such is the case with the Writing Attitude Survey. These constructs were operationalized by defining the construct and its domains and developing items and **response scales** consistent with the construct and its domains.

Constructs that are made up of a single domain require fewer items, such is the case with only 10 items comprising the scale Teacher and Literacy Coach Exposure/Opportunity to Benefit. When a construct consists of multiple domains, then more items are necessary, as is the case for the Cultural Attitudes and Climate Questionnaire with 10 domains and 100 items.

Assisting you in defining the construct is the completion of a literature review. A literature review contributes to your learning the language associated with the phenomenon of interest. The literature review also will help you to more precisely define your construct. For example, revisit the two scales in Table 1.2 that are measuring respondents' attitude toward diversity. The scales, Attitudes toward Diversity Scale (ADS) and Cultural Attitudes and Climate Questionnaire (CACQ), both claim to measure attitudes toward diversity. Examination of the subscales, however, shows that the ADS scale measures three aspects of attitudes toward diversity in the workplace, whereas the CACQ scale measures 10 different aspects of diversity on a university campus. Thus, a literature review assists in clearly defining the constructs that are associated with your research study or program evaluation.

Extending from the literature review will be the development of a **conceptual framework**. A framework specifies the relationships between the constructs within a phenomenon. In specifying the relationships among the constructs, the framework provides a context for the survey scale that a researcher will adopt or develop for a study. The conceptual framework consists of a **narrative** and a **model**. The narrative defines and describes the constructs in the framework and makes explicit the relationships between the constructs in the study. The conceptual model is a diagram that commonly uses circles and arrows to depict the proposed links among a set of constructs thought to be related to a specific problem. Together the narrative and model frame the constructs and relationships that comprise the phenomenon of interest (i.e., research focus) that is the focus of one's study. To continue our example with the construct of student engagement, we might use the results from the literature review to specify whether the domains of academic and social engagement influence one another and whether they influence student achievement. Chapter 3 focuses on the development of conceptual frameworks.

Review Potential Instruments

In the previous section, we indicated that a researcher or an evaluator will adopt or develop a scale for a study. Before you commit to the development of a new survey scale, a review of published instruments will be beneficial. Developing a new survey scale is time consuming and expensive. If an instrument is available and it meets your research needs, then consider adopting or adapting the scale. Not all instruments, however, are of good quality. Thus, Chapter 2 provides guidance in the review process. Even if you do not adopt or adapt an instrument, the experience of reviewing potential scales will expose you to the language used by researchers in the field, provide examples of how other researchers operationalized the construct, and deepen your understanding of the phenomenon of interest.

Write Items and Response Scales

As shown in Figure 1.3, a next step in the survey process is the development of survey items and response scales. The constructs that you included in your conceptual framework will be the focus of item development. For a study related to student engagement, items must be written for the domains of academic engagement and social engagement. The items in Figure 1.4 are closed response; that is, survey participants read an item and then choose their answer from a set of options. These options consist of numerical and/ or verbal descriptors. For example, in Figure 1.4, the first item is "As a

TABLE 1.2. Examples of Constructs and Their Domains

Title of the scale/instrument	Construct measured	Domains/subscales	Operationalization
Attitudes toward Diversity Scale (Montei, Adams, & Eggers, 1996)	Attitude toward diversity in the work environment	1. Attitude toward minority coworkers 2. Attitude toward minority supervisor 3. Attitude toward hiring and promoting of minorities	30 items with 5-point, Likert-type response scales: Strongly agree to Strongly disagree.
Caregiver Survey (Morgan, Sherlock, & Ritchie, 2010)	Job satisfaction	1. Job satisfaction 2. Supervisory relationships 3. Job environment	15 items with 5-point, Likert-type response scales: Very dissatisfied to Very satisfied.
Cultural Attitudes and Climate Questionnaire (Helm, Sedlacek, & Prieto, 1998)[a]	Attitudes toward diversity and overall satisfaction	1. Racial tension—perception and experience of racial conflict on campus 2. Cross-cultural comfort—comfort with racially ethnically similar and dissimilar faculty and peers 3. Diversity awareness—sensitivity to racial–ethnic differences 4. Racial pressures—pressure to conform to racial–ethnic stereotypes 5. Residence hall tension—perception of interracial and interethnic conflict in residence halls	100 items with 5-point, Likert-type response scales: Strongly agree to Strongly disagree.
Ethical Assessment Practices (Johnson, Green, Kim, & Pope, 2008)	Perceptions about the ethics of classroom assessment practices	1. Bias/fairness 2. Communication about grading 3. Confidentiality 4. Grading practices 5. Multiple assessment opportunities 6. Standardized test preparation 7. Test administration	36 items with 2-point response scales: Ethical and Unethical.

10

Instrument (source)	Domain	Subscales	Format
Index of Teaching Stress (Abidin, Greene, & Konold, 2003)	Teacher stress	1. Attention-deficit/hyperactivity disorder 2. Student characteristics: Emotional Lability/Low Adaptability, Anxiety/Withdrawal, Low Ability/ Learning Disability, and Aggressiveness/Conduct Disorder 3. Teacher characteristics: Sense of Competence/ Need for Support, Loss of Satisfaction from Teaching, Disruption of the Teaching Process, and Frustration Working with Parents	90 items with 5-point response scales: Never stressful to Very often stressful; Never distressing to Very distressing.
Motivation to Read Profile: The Reading Survey (Gambrell, Palmer, Codling, & Mazzoni, 1996)	Student reading motivation	1. Self-concept as a reader 2. Value of reading	20 items with 4-point response scales.
Portfolio Assessment Review (Johnson, 1996)	Artifacts useful in determining levels of family literacy	No subscales	15 items in a checklist format.
Student Survey on High School Transition (Johnson, Davis, Fisher, Johnson, & Somerindyke, 2000)	Student engagement	Academic engagement Social engagement	17 items with 4-point response scales: Never to All the time; Strongly disagree to Strongly agree.
Teacher and Literacy Coach Exposure/Opportunity to Benefit (Office of Program Evaluation/South Carolina Educational Policy Center, 2005)	Benefits from interactions with the literacy coach	No subscales	10 items with 4-point response scales: Never to Often.
Writing Attitude Survey (Kear, Coffman, McKenna, & Ambrosio, 2000)	Attitude toward writing	No subscales	28 items with 4-point response scales: Very happy to Very upset.

[a]The Cultural Attitudes and Climate Questionnaire has 10 domains. We show five of the domains.

11

ninth-grade student I enjoy learning new things." The response scale for the item consists of numerical ratings (i.e., 1–4) and verbal descriptors (i.e., "Rarely" to "All the time"). The item-writing guidelines in Chapters 4 and 5 assist in writing items and response scales that will be clear to survey respondents and provide information that will support researchers in drawing accurate conclusions.

Format Survey and Determine the Administration Method

In determining the format of the survey, it is important to consider the method of administration and any special considerations for formatting items within the survey instrument. Formats of self-administered surveys include **questionnaires** completed individually or in group settings, mail surveys, and web pages. Other options to consider include face-to-face and telephone interviews as well as focus groups. In Chapter 6, we present qualities to inform your selection in determining the method for your survey administration.

Submit the Survey Scale for Review

Developing a survey requires a great deal of time and financial resources. In order for this investment to "pay off," the survey scale should be reviewed to correct any flaws that would negate survey results. Various reviews that will contribute to the quality of your survey scales include feedback from subject matter experts, a survey methodologist, a copyeditor, and a diversity committee. In Chapter 6, we expand on the contributions that each of these reviewers offers.

Avoiding critical flaws also requires piloting the survey with a group of respondents who are similar to those who will complete the final instrument. This select group of respondents both completes the survey instrument (e.g., web page or paper-and-pencil questionnaire) and provides feedback about the items. In Chapter 6, we discuss the types of information that a small pilot can provide.

Field Test the Instrument and Investigate Item and Scale Quality

A final task in developing a survey instrument is to conduct a **field test** that is large enough to allow statistical analyses to determine if the items and scales have adequate statistical qualities (see Chapter 8). On the completion of this review, any final changes should be made and the survey instrument is ready for use.

Document the Development of the Survey Scale

Part of the development of a survey scale is the documentation of the instrument construction and the technical information related to item quality, **reliability**, and **validity** evidence (American Educational Research Association [AERA], American Psychological Association [APA], & National Council on Measurement in Education [NCME], 2014). This documentation might serve as the description of the instrumentation in the *Method* section of a research article, a dissertation, an evaluation report, or a technical report. Preparation of the documentation for your scale requires consideration of the methods best suited for informing the readers of your findings. As we describe in Chapter 10, tables and graphs have the potential to contribute to the documentation process. In this instance, if properly constructed, tables and graphs can facilitate the communication of the quality of the instrument.

Attitudes, Knowledge, and Behaviors

At this point you might ask, "So, what constructs can I investigate using surveys?" Often, researchers develop survey scales to measure respondents' attitudes, knowledge, or behaviors.

Attitudes

Various terms have been used to describe the term "attitude." Matwin and Fabrigar (2007) wrote, "An attitude is a relatively general and enduring evaluation of a person, object, or concept along a **dimension** ranging from positive to negative" (p. 53). Others more broadly defined the construct of attitude to include opinions, beliefs, feelings, intents, preferences, stands, and values (Crespi, 1971; Fink, 2002; Nardi, 2003; Ostrom, 1971; Schuman & Presser, 1996). What these terms have in common with the construct of attitude is their evaluative nature. Attitude items measure respondents' evaluations of an attitude object (Fazio & Olson, 2007; Kyriakidou, 2009; Schwarz, Knäuper, Oyserman, & Stich, 2008). Ostrom (1971, p. 593) stated, "The measurement of attitude involves locating the individual's 'typical' response toward the attitude object on an evaluative continuum." In the Writing Attitude Survey (Kear, Coffman, McKenna, & Ambrosio, 2000, p. 17), for example, the attitude object is writing and uses such statements as:

> How would you feel writing a letter stating your opinion about a topic?
> How would you feel writing poetry for fun?

The response scale for each item forms an evaluative continuum that ranges from very happy, to somewhat happy, to somewhat upset, and to very upset.

Items that measure attitude are typically composed of how respondents feel (e.g., "Favorable"–"Unfavorable") and how strongly they feel (e.g., "Very unfavorable"–"Very favorable"). These items often use an agreement scale (e.g., "Disagree"–"Agree"). To gauge respondents' attitudes requires the development of a set of statements that express positive or negative stands toward an attitude object, such as the quality of service at their physician's office (Matwin & Fabrigar, 2007).

Knowledge

On occasion, researchers want to gauge study participants' knowledge about a topic. Knowledge can be conceptualized as how much respondents know about an issue or their familiarity with a topic (Nardi, 2003). That is, knowledgeable respondents are informed about a topic (Fowler, 1995).

Knowledge items in a survey play an important role in that they can be used to determine if potential respondents have enough knowledge for the researcher to ask their opinion about a topic (Fink, 2003). These types of items allow a researcher to mark the study participants' responses as correct or incorrect and calculate the number correct to indicate the extent of the survey participants' understanding.

Questions that gauge participant understanding about a topic can serve to identify gaps in knowledge for awareness campaigns. For example, a survey on breast cancer can serve the purpose of identifying misconceptions that should be addressed in an awareness campaign. Below are two true–false items that gauge survey respondents' understanding of breast cancer.

1. Early detection of breast cancer is the key to successful treatment.
5. Women who drink more than one alcoholic beverage a day increase their risk for breast cancer.

(University of Rochester Medical Center, 2014)

Knowledge-based items also can be used to explain attitudes and behaviors. To continue the breast cancer example, a researcher might investigate whether respondents' understanding predicts their likelihood of having a breast examination.

One consideration is which type of item format—true–false, matching, or multiple-choice—is appropriate for use in a survey scale that measures knowledge. It is doubtful that study participants are likely to answer items that look like a test; so we rule out the use of multiple-choice questions in a survey.

Another possibility is the true–false item format and its variations (Fowler, 1995; Orcher, 2007). On the Internet one often sees web pages about myths associated with a health condition. The previous items about breast cancer are from such websites. Fairly nonthreatening, these questions do not have the feel of a test and offer the potential for gauging survey respondents' level of knowledge. We explore this type of item in Chapters 4 and 5.

Behaviors

Behaviors are the actions in which respondents engage. Put simply, behaviors are what people do (Fink, 2003; Nardi, 2003). Survey items that address behaviors are concerned with time, duration, and frequency (Fink, 2003). A distinction should be made: Self-reported behaviors are not the same as observation. In *Survey Scales*, we focus on the use of surveys to collect self-reported information about behaviors.

Key Qualities of a Survey Scale: Reliability and Validity

By reliability, we mean the consistency of respondents' scores across such conditions as items and occasions. In other words, reliability addresses whether a respondent's score would be consistent if she were to complete the survey on a different occasion or complete different items. Survey participants' responses change somewhat from one occasion to another. Also, we understand that a respondent might be presented with items that focus on an area in which she has little knowledge; however, if different survey items had been selected for the scale, then the content might be familiar to the respondent and she would respond differently. To remediate such circumstances, survey developers include multiple items in a scale. Return to the Student Engagement Scale in Figure 1.4. We included seven items to measure the construct of Social Engagement. Relying on one item, such as "As a ninth-grade student I talk with adults (teachers, counselors, coaches) when I have problems," might result in an inappropriate decision about a student's engagement.

The concept of validity is associated with accuracy (Kane, 1982; Stallings & Gillmore, 1971). That is, validity addresses the accuracy of our inferences (e.g., decisions) based on our interpretation of the scores from the survey scales. In other words, based on the scores from the survey scale, are we likely to make accurate (i.e., valid) decisions about respondents? For example, will we make valid decisions about respondents' understanding of breast cancer? If the website was not vetted by experts in the field and critical information about breast cancer was omitted, then any interpretations of respondents' knowledge would be inaccurate (i.e., not valid).

Throughout the remainder of *Survey Scales*, we revisit the issues of reliability and validity as they apply to writing items, selecting response scales, completing item- and scale-level analyses to select items, and determining the number of items for the scale and its subscales. We will revisit reliability and validity to illustrate the effect of each on the consistency of scores and the accuracy of decisions, respectively, based on those scores. Why the intense focus on these qualities of survey scales? The procedures outlined in *Survey Scales* are potential sources of validity evidence. Developers of surveys should both (1) follow such rigorous procedures in their survey development and (2) document them as part of the validity evidence associated with the survey scale.

As we mentioned earlier, developing a new survey scale is demanding. So prior to committing energy and resources to constructing a new scale, a review of existing scales is useful. Examining survey scales published in research articles and reading critiques in the literature benefit a researcher in identifying a preexisting survey scale that meets his or her research needs. In Chapter 2, we discuss available resources for reviewing published instruments and the qualities for guiding the selection of instrumentation for your study.

FURTHER READING

Fink, A. (2017). *How to conduct surveys: A step-by-step guide* (6th ed.). Thousand Oaks, CA: Sage.

> *Outlines the steps in conducting a survey. Provides rules for writing items and examples to illustrate the application of the rules.*

Fowler, F. (2014). *Survey research methods* (5th ed.). Thousand Oaks, CA: Sage.

> *Provides an in-depth discussion of conducting a survey. Discusses issues related to the development of survey questions.*

CHAPTER EXERCISES

1. Describe a survey that you completed. Include the purpose of the survey and its characteristics that lead you to conclude its purpose.

2. What type of item (checklists, true–false variations, or Likert-style items) comprises the scale in Figure 1.4?

3. Are the items closed-response or open-response?

4. Write another statement that could be added to the Academic Engagement subscale.

5. Write a statement that could be added to the Social Engagement subscale.

   a. How are these two items different?
   b. How are these two items the same?

6. After reviewing a draft of a student's survey scale, the dissertation chair noted that a section on items related to interpersonal relationships needed to be added. Is this an issue of reliability or validity? Justify your answer.

CHAPTER 2

Adopting or Adapting an Existing Scale

. . . before developing your own measure for research or practice, you should consider searching for one that has already been developed and is suitable for your purposes.

—GALL, GALL, AND BORG (2010, p. 142)

Introduction

Constructing a survey scale is a demanding process; many writers in educational research therefore recommend that prior to developing a scale, researchers and evaluators should review existing instruments for possible adoption or adaptation. In this chapter, we discuss conducting a search to locate instruments and introduce resources that provide critiques of existing measurement tools such as attitude scales. Given that existing scales do not always address the needs for one's study, we also provide guidance on the extent to which a researcher can appropriately incorporate items or sections of a published survey scale into his or her instrument and on the need to obtain permission to use copyrighted scales.

Reviewing Potential Instruments for Adoption or Adaptation

What steps should one take to locate potential scales to incorporate into a survey? Nitko (n.d.) outlined the following steps in the evaluation of an instrument:

1. Clarify the purpose of the instrument.
2. Use your research context in evaluating an instrument.

3. Review journal articles and professional critiques of the instrument.
4. Obtain copies of the instrument you are evaluating.
5. Summarize the strengths and weaknesses of the instrument.
6. Make a decision about the instrument and support that decision.

We discuss each step in the sections below.

Clarify the Instrument's Purpose

A critical first step is to clarify (1) the purpose of obtaining information (i.e., data) from survey respondents and (2) the use of the information for decision making. Clarity about purpose helps to select an instrument that provides information contributing to valid inferences (e.g., decisions, conclusions, predictions). Examples of instrument purposes include (1) determining client satisfaction with services, (2) assessing student attitudes toward science, and (3) gaining subject matter experts' feedback about critical knowledge, skills, and abilities for a licensure examination.

Consider the Research Context

In determining which instrument is appropriate for your research study or program evaluation, in terms of your research context consider the data that are already available. For example, school climate data might be available from a climate survey administered annually by a state department of education. Duplicating items from a state climate survey in your instrument might raise the issue of respecting the survey participants' time.

Review Journal Articles and Critiques

A next step is to locate and review journal articles and professional critiques of instruments. Articles about instruments can be located by searching such resources as ERIC, Education Source, PsycINFO, and Google Scholar. For example, a search using the term "attitude toward diversity" in Google Scholar produced an article about diversity in the *Journal of College Counseling*. The article "The Relationship between Attitudes toward Diversity and Overall Satisfaction of University Students by Race" (Helm, Sedlacek, & Prieto, 1998) includes the instrument items in an appendix. A review of the items helps one to examine the fit between Helm et al.'s instrument and your research focus. A review of the items in the instrument also allows you to begin to see how others operationalize the construct of "attitude toward diversity."

Professional journals are a source for descriptions and critiques of instruments. For example, *The Reading Teacher* published articles about the Elementary Reading Attitude Survey (McKenna & Kear, 1999) and the Writing Attitude Survey (WAS; Kear et al., 2000). Descriptions of instruments are also included in some articles published in the journal *Educational and Psychological Measurement*. Similarly, the authors of articles on the website *Practical Assessment, Research and Evaluation* describe instruments used in research studies.

The website the *Test Collection at ETS* contains a database with over 25,000 instruments. The *Test Collection* provides a record view that includes the title of the instrument, the author's name, the availability (i.e., address of publisher or ETS weblink for purchase), the year of publication, major and minor descriptors (e.g., stress variables, Likert scale), and an abstract. As an example, the abstract for the Index of Teaching Stress (Abidin, Greene, & Konold, 2003) reads:

> The Index of Teaching Stress (ITS) measures the stress teachers experience by way of their interactions with specific students. There are 90 items answered on a 5-point Likert-style rating scale. It takes approximately 20–25 minutes to complete the survey. ITS is appropriate for use with teachers from preschool through grade 12. Technical information is provided. (Educational Testing Service, 2014, para. 1)

Another resource, the *Mental Measurements Yearbook*, provides critiques of published standardized instruments that assess attitudes, behaviors, and achievement. Each yearbook provides critiques of standardized instruments published since the previous issue. In addition to providing descriptive information, typically two reviewers critique each instrument. The value of these critiques in determining the quality of an instrument warrants a closer examination of the *Mental Measurements Yearbook*; so we revisit this resource later in the chapter.

Request Copies of Instruments

After reading the reviews of instruments, you should request review copies of the instruments that appear suitable for adopting. These instruments are the authors' operationalization of the construct. In the review set, the publisher should provide descriptions of the instrument content and a rationale behind its selection; materials related to scoring, reporting, and interpreting instrument results; the cost of the materials and scoring; and technical information (e.g., reliability and validity) about the instrument (Nitko, n.d.).

Summarize Strengths and Weaknesses

For each instrument being considered for adoption, develop a list of strengths and weaknesses. Nitko (n.d.) advised that the review of the instruments should be completed by a committee. Such will be the case if the instrument will be used to collect data for an evaluation to make decisions about a program in a school district. The committee's members should be representative of those who will be completing the instrument and those who will be using the data. In the case of a school district, the stakeholders might include teachers, principals, parents, and school board members.

In considering adoption of an instrument for evaluation or practitioner purposes, it might be beneficial to use subcommittees in the initial review of instruments' strengths and weaknesses. Qualities to consider are listed in the review sheet in Figure 2.1. The review sheet provides a framework for the evaluation of an instrument. The first column lists the qualities of an instrument, and the second column provides a place for recording information that will inform a decision about the instrument. The third and fourth columns provide a place for the reviewer to indicate if the quality is acceptable for adopting the instrument.

Committee members with subject matter expertise could focus on review of the content section. Those practitioners who will use the instrument results can provide feedback about the usefulness of the results for professional practice and they can address the section on practical evaluation. A technical evaluation committee could summarize information on validity and reliability. Selection of an instrument for research purposes can be informed by members of a committee with skills in measurement and survey design.

Make a Decision about the Instrument

In preparation for making a decision about an instrument to adopt, in the instance of evaluators and practitioners the subcommittees mentioned earlier would report to the committee of the whole. This step provides all committee members with the same information and allows questions to be asked. Then, either by consensus or by vote, a final recommendation should be made by the committee. In the instance of a research team, the decision should be informed by discussion among the subject matter experts and measurement and survey specialists.

The *Mental Measurements Yearbook*: A Source for Reviews of Instruments

A valued resource that provides critiques of instruments is the *Mental Measurements Yearbook* (MMY). The MMY provides reviews that assist you in making judgments about the quality of an instrument (Nitko, 2014). The instruments in the yearbook are organized alphabetically. In the back of each volume are a series of indices that assist you in locating a critique

Name of Instrument: _____ Date: _____ Reviewer: _____

	Notes	Acceptable	Not Acceptable
Content Evaluation			
1. Publisher's description and rationale for including the items in the instrument.			
2. Quality of the items.			
3. Currency of the content measured by the items on the instrument.			
4. Match of the content of the instrument items to the evaluation or the research focus.			
5. The extent to which the items are inclusive and attend to diversity.			
Usefulness of the Results for Professional Practice			
1. Publisher's description and rationale for how the instrument results may be used by practitioners, evaluators, or researchers.			
2. Evaluators' and practitioners' evaluations of how they could use the instrument results to improve practice or researchers' justifications of how they can use the instrument to study research questions.			
3. Overlap of the proposed instrument with the tools currently used by evaluators, practitioners, or researchers.			
Technical Evaluation			
1. Representativeness, recency, and local relevance of the national norms (if applicable).			
2. Types of reliability coefficients and their values (use range of values for each type if necessary).			

3. Summary of the empirical evidence for the validity associated with the test for the specific purpose(s) you have in mind for the instrument.	
4. Likelihood that using the scores from the proposed instrument will be used in a way that has adverse effects on persons with disabilities, minority group members, or gender groups.	
Practical Evaluation	
1. Quality of the manual and other materials.	
2. Ease of administration and scoring.	
3. Cost and usefulness of scoring services.	
4. Estimated costs (time and money) if the instrument is adopted.	
5. Likely reaction of the public if the instrument is adopted for (a) evaluator or practitioner purposes or (b) peer reviewers if adopted for research purposes.	
Overall Evaluation	
1. Evaluative comments on published reviews (e.g., MMY).	
2. Your evaluative conclusions about the positive aspects of the instrument.	
3. Your evaluative conclusions about the negative aspects of the instrument.	
4. Your summary and recommendations about adopting this instrument for each of the specific purposes intended for the research study or evaluation.	

FIGURE 2.1. An evaluation guide for reviewing an instrument. Adapted from Nitko (n.d.) with permission of the publisher, Buros Center for Testing, *www.buros.org*. Copyright © 2014 Buros Center for Testing.

23

of an instrument. An index of titles provides an alphabetical list of titles of instruments with an entry number that gives the location in the MMY for each title. Occasionally, an instrument is known by its acronym, such as WISC-R, also known as the Wechsler Intelligence Scale for Children. Thus, each volume also includes an index that provides an alphabetical list of acronyms. If you do not know the title of an instrument that measures the construct of interest in your study, then an important index is the Classified Subject Index. In this index, the MMY classifies instruments into one of 18 major categories: Achievement, Behavior Assessment, Development, Education, English and Language, Fine Arts, Foreign Languages, Intelligence and General Aptitude, Mathematics, Miscellaneous, Neuropsychological, Personality, Reading, Science, Sensory-Motor, Social Studies, Speech and Hearing, and Vocations. Other indices include a list of publishers and their addresses, names (i.e., test authors, reviewers, and authors cited in the review), and scores (e.g., Concern for Others, Critical Thinking, Hyperactivity).

Elements of a critique include the test entry,[1] description, development, technical qualities, reviewer commentary, and a summary. In this section, we use Mildred Murray-Ward's review (2007) of the Index of Teaching Stress (Abidin et al., 2003) to illustrate the parts of a review.

Test Entry

The test entry includes descriptive information about the instrument, such as the title of the test, the authors of the instrument, its purpose, the targeted **population** for which the instrument is intended, scores provided by the test, and time allotted for administration (see Figure 2.2). The test entry section is prepared by the staff and editors of the MMY (Nitko, 2014). A quick review of information in the test entry allows you to determine if (1) the purpose of the instrument is consistent with your evaluation or research study, (2) the target population for the preexisting survey is compatible with the target population for your study, (3) the scales will provide the types of scores needed, and (4) the cost of using the instrument is within your budget. Key descriptive information about the Index of Teaching Stress includes the following: (1) the authors are Abidin, Greene, and Konold (2003); (2) the purpose of the instrument is to assess the relation between student behavior and a teacher's stress level; (3) teachers comprise the target population; and (4) the types of domain scores produced include a Total Stress Score; Attention-Deficit/Hyperactivity Disorder; Student Characteristics; and Emotional Lability/Low Adaptability.

---

[1] The MMY refers to instruments as tests; however, the instruments included in a Yearbook extend to measures of attitudes and behaviors. We use the term "instrument" when not directly quoting the MMY.

Title:	Index of Teaching Stress.
Acronyms:	ITS.
Authors:	Abidin, Richard R.; Greene, Ross W.; Konold, Timothy R.
Publication Date:	2003–2004.
Publisher Information:	Psychological Assessment Resources, Inc., 16204 N. Florida Avenue, Lutz, FL 33549-8119; Telephone: 800-331-8378; FAX: 800-727-9329; E-mail: custsupp@parinc.com; Web: www.parinc.com.
Purpose:	Designed to assess the effects of a specific student's behavior on a teacher's stress level and self-perception.
Test Category:	Education.
Administration:	Group.
Population:	Teachers from preschool to 12th grade.
Scores:	Total Stress Score; Attention-Deficit/Hyperactivity Disorder; Student Characteristics; Emotional Lability/Low Adaptability; Anxiety/Withdrawal; Low Ability/Learning Disability; Aggressive/Conduct Disorder; Teacher Characteristics; Sense of Competence/Need for Support; Loss of Satisfaction from Teaching; Disruption of the Teaching Process; Frustration Working with Parents.
Time:	20–25 minutes.
Price:	2007: $134 per introductory kit including manual (2004, 89 pages), 25 reusable item booklets, 25 answer sheets, and 25 profile forms.
Number of Reviews:	1.
Reviewer:	Murray-Ward, Mildred (California State University Stanislaus).
Cross Reference:	For a review by Mildred Murray-Ward, see 17:88.
Yearbook:	17.
Record Source:	*Mental Measurements Yearbook with Tests in Print.*
Accession Number:	TIP17033224.
Mental Measurements Review Number:	17033224.
Database:	*Mental Measurements Yearbook with Tests in Print.*

(continued)

FIGURE 2.2. A critique from the MMY. Copyright © 2014 Buros Center for Testing. Reprinted by permission.

Review of the Index of Teaching Stress by MILDRED MURRAY-WARD, Dean, College of Education, California State University, Stanislaus, Turlock, CA:

DESCRIPTION. The Index of Teaching Stress (ITS) is a unique instrument that measures teacher stress in relation to interactions with students. Unlike other instruments that measure teacher stress by focusing on global measures of job satisfaction, the ITS focuses on specific student behaviors and teachers' specific feelings of self-efficacy as a teacher in the student–teacher relationship.

The primary purpose of the ITS is to measure teacher stress experienced through interactions with a specific student. The authors state that the ITS allows assessment of students and provides data for consultation with teachers to maximize teacher effectiveness with a specific child. Indeed, the last section of the manual contains suggestions for clinical and research applications. The manual also provides profiles or case studies presenting score profiles and interpretations of results. In addition, the authors claim that through this assessment process teacher stress may be reduced, teacher objectivity could be increased, and teacher–student relationships could be enhanced.

The target group for whom the instrument is intended is composed of teachers in preschool to 12th grade in regular or special education classroom settings.

The instrument is composed of 90 statements, organized through careful development and analysis into three scales. The first is the Attention-Deficit/Hyperactivity Disorder Domain composed of 16 items. Second is the Student Characteristics Domain (31 items), including the following scales: Emotional Lability/Low Adaptability, Anxiety/Withdrawal, Low Ability/Learning Disability, and Aggressiveness/Conduct Disorder. Third, the Teacher Characteristics Domain is composed of 43 items, including the following scales: Sense of Competence/Need for Support, Loss of Satisfaction from Teaching, Disruption of the Teaching Process, and Frustration Working with Parents.

Respondents use two different 5-point response scales. For Part A, respondents choose from: 1–Never Stressful to 5–Very Often Stressful. For Part B, respondents use: 1–Never Distressing to 5–Very Distressing.

DEVELOPMENT. The ITS was developed based on a model of Teaching Stress initially designed in 1989 in response to the need for a teacher stress instrument comparable to the Parenting Stress Index (Abidin, 1983, 1995). The model uses six understandings of human behavior:

> (a) recognition that temperament plays a major dispositional role in exhibited behavior; (b) attachment style and interpersonal relationships are both motivational sources and moderators of disposition; (c) cultural and social skills are factors that influence the expression and interpretation of behavior; (d) behavior is learned, shaped, and influenced by behavioral factors ranging from cues to reinforcements; (e) human behavioral and emotional responses are both produced and moderated by perceptions and cognitions; and (f) behavior is embedded in social and physical contexts that influence behavioral expression, cognitions, and emotions. (professional manual, p. 2).

The ITS was created from a strong theoretical foundation clearly explained in the professional manual. The items were created through examination of the impact of students on teacher behavior and teachers' attitude toward self. The authors claim that the instrument is unique in that it focuses on students and their relationship to teacher stress and not other occupational factors that may contribute to teacher stress levels.

(continued)

FIGURE 2.2. *(continued)*

The authors created the 90-item instrument by first conducting focus groups with teachers who reported student characteristics, thoughts about themselves, and school contexts. A total of 108 items were generated from the information obtained from the focus groups. The 108 items were reduced to 90 and factor analyzed into two scales. The authors clearly described this process and their rationale for technical decisions, including the reasoning behind establishing a separate ADHD scale.

TECHNICAL. Standardization. Technical qualities of the ITS are clearly discussed in the manual. The final instrument was normed on a sample of 814 teachers who rated randomly selected students. The teachers ranged from 1 to 41 (mean of 14.0) years of experience, with the majority in regular classrooms (16.4% in special education classrooms). The students ranged from ages 5 to 18 years (mean of 10.9). The teachers and students were matched to the most recent U.S. Census and included teachers from Georgia, Massachusetts, New York, Texas, and Virginia. Student characteristics were matched to 1995 NCES data on student populations.

The 674 teachers who rated students with specifically identified behavior problems had a mean of 13.7 years of experience, with 17.3% in special education classrooms. The rated students were from 5 to 18 (mean 10.2) years of age. It was not clear whether there was any overlap in the group of teachers who rated randomly selected students and those with specific behavior problems. Again, the group selected was matched to 1995 NCES data.

Normative scores include percentiles and T-scores. The authors also looked at possible grade-level effects on ratings and found no significant differences in ratings of students from three different grade levels.

The authors recommend choosing the Randomly Selected Student Sample norms when determining teachers' scores relative to other teachers, child study, and in case consultation and other clinical situations. The authors recommend using both sets of norms to illustrate findings such as comparing teacher scores with those teachers who also teach behavior problem students, and in gauging the relative severity of the classroom situation.

Reliability. Both internal consistency and test–retest reliability of the ITS were examined. Internal consistency reliability alpha coefficients exceeded .90 for the ITS domains and Total score for the Behavior Problem Student and Randomly Selected Student samples. Test–retest reliability was estimated with 42 white teachers' ratings of the same Behavior Problem Students using a 1-month interval. Reliabilities ranged from .30 to .70 for the domains, .57 for Student Characteristics, .70 for Teacher Characteristics, and .65 for Total Stress. The reliability studies provide evidence that the instrument is internally consistent and moderately sensitive to "episodic" student behavior.

Validity. In the area of validity, the authors established the content validity of the items through the use of teacher focus groups and using the responses to generate ITS items. The authors also explored discriminant and concurrent validity. The discriminant validity studies revealed that the scores were not related to general stress of teachers. In addition, the scores are sensitive to intervention and positively related to teacher ratings of likelihood of the student being referred for services. Concurrent validity studies indicated that scores on the ITS are positively related to the students' social skills, and negatively related to the quality of the teacher–student relationship. Interestingly, female teachers were more stressed with male students and male teachers were more stressed with female students.

(continued)

FIGURE 2.2. *(continued)*

COMMENTARY. The ITS is a unique and interesting instrument that may help in assessing teacher–student relationships. It serves a vital need in examining student-related stress in teachers that could impact classroom interactions and resulting learning environments. The instrument has several strengths. First, it possesses a strong theoretical foundation and research base. Second, the technical qualities and processes of development appear excellent. Of particular note are the studies establishing content validity and the procedures used to develop the scales. The authors were also careful to examine cutscore ranges that could trigger intervention.

Although the instrument does possess excellent qualities, there are some weaknesses and notes of caution. First, although the authors clearly discuss the application of the Randomly Selected Student Sample, they do not provide as clear directions on use of the Behavior Problem Student Sample. In addition, the authors provide some interesting case studies using profiles of teachers and specific students. Although these are interesting examples, the profiles include interpretation of scores and accompanying actions not validated in previous studies. Because these cases are not based on empirical studies, the reader is cautioned not to over-interpret the scale scores.

SUMMARY. The ITS is a high-quality instrument designed to examine teacher stress levels. The instrument is an important addition to the field because teacher stress can impact the quality of the learning environment and, therefore, the learning potential for students. The authors' careful attention to instrument development make it an excellent tool in forming an understanding of student–teacher interaction as information used in part to generate student interventions. As with any instrument, this reviewer recommends the use of multiple data sources. Therefore, when using the ITS, additional data on classroom environment should be collected and considered in making such determinations.

REVIEWER'S REFERENCES

Abidin, R. R. (1983). *Parenting Stress Index*. Charlottesville, VA: Pediatric Psychology Press.
Abidin, R. R. (1995). *Parenting Stress Index: Professional manual* (3rd ed.). Odessa, FL: Psychological Assessment Resources.

FIGURE 2.2. *(continued)*

The remaining sections of a critique are written by an external reviewer. The reviewer's critique is based on his or her evaluation of the materials (e.g., the instrument, answer sheets, and technical manual) submitted by the authors of the instrument.

Description

In the description section, the reviewer discusses the instrument's purpose(s), identifies the population, describes the content, and identifies the intended uses. Also, the reviewer provides a summary about the administration of the instrument, the scores, and the scoring. In the case of the Index of Teaching Stress (ITS), Murray-Ward (2007) stated the purpose of the instrument and contrasted (1) its focus on teacher stress in relation to interaction with students and (2) instruments that measure teacher stress in terms of global measures of job satisfaction. She provided additional information about the types of domain scores—Attention-Deficit/Hyperactivity Disorder, Student Characteristics, and Teacher Characteristics—and the number of items in each domain. Murray-Ward further explained the relation between domain scores and scale scores. For example, the Teacher Characteristics domain consists of Sense of Competence/Need for Support, Loss of Satisfaction from Teaching; Disruption of the Teaching Process; and Frustration Working with Parents. She also noted that the items used 5-point response scales.

Development

The reviewer's discussion of the ITS development includes a description of the **theory** that underlies the construct that the instrument is intended to measure, the method for development of the items to measure the construct, and the theoretical reasoning and empirical information about item functioning that guided selection of the final set of items (Nitko, 2014). Murray-Ward (2007) wrote that a strength of the instrument development was its basis in a strong theoretical foundation. She also commented on the use of focus groups to identify relevant student characteristics, teachers' thoughts about themselves, and school contexts as related to stress.

Technical Qualities

In the technical section, the reviewer considers the psychometric properties of the instrument. This includes information about standardization (norming sample), types of reliability evidence (e.g., **internal consistency**, test–retest), and validity evidence. In the review of the Index of Teaching Stress, Murray-Ward wrote about the norming of the instrument. The norming involved a **sample** of 814 teachers (i.e., the norming group for the ITS). These teachers completed the instrument, and their scores provide a comparison for teachers who subsequently complete the Index of Teaching Stress. For example, when a teacher takes the ITS, one might ask if his Total Score is higher than the **mean** of the norming group, lower than the mean, or at the mean. In her review, Murray-Ward also considered the reliability (i.e., consistency) of the scores and the validity evidence that the authors of the instrument collected to support the decisions about teacher stress that were to be made from the scores.

Reviewer Commentary

In the commentary section, the reviewer addresses the instrument's strengths and weaknesses and considers the adequacy of the theoretic model supporting instrument use. According to Murray-Ward (2007), the strengths included the strong theoretical background, technical qualities, and the development procedures. The reviewer, however, raises questions about the use of case studies with profiles of teachers and students to demonstrate the interpretation of scores and accompanying actions. Murray-Ward expresses caution because the cases were not validated.

Summary

In the summary section, the reviewer provides conclusions and recommendations about the quality of the instrument. Murray-Ward (2007) describes the value of the instrument in examining teacher stress levels. She also revisits the issue of the quality of instrument development.

Plagiarism and Copyright Infringement

After your review of existing instruments, you will decide to adopt, adapt, or develop your own scale. Adopting or adapting an instrument requires you to obtain permission from the holder of the copyright to use the scale in your study and subsequent publications. Adapting involves modifying a scale by retaining the original items suited to your study, deleting items that are not relevant to your study, revising items to be consistent with the scale purpose, and developing new items to fill in the gaps in the scale. In producing a new scale, you will develop items original to your instrument. You also might decide to include a few of the items from the different scales that you reviewed. Whether adopting an instrument, adapting a scale, or developing a new scale, you want to avoid plagiarism of works and copyright infringement. Although these terms are often used in tandem, they are two different ethical issues (Baker, 2013; Fishman, 2011).

Plagiarism

An author has plagiarized a work when he or she presents the words or ideas of another as if the work were his or her own (APA, 2010; Baker, 2013). Stated another way, "A plagiarist is a person who poses as the *originator* of words he did not write, ideas he did not conceive, or facts he did not discover" (Fishman, 2011, p. 278). Following APA writing guidelines can help prevent plagiarism. Thus, the developer of an instrument can attribute work to the original author through the use of quotation marks to indicate the use of the exact words of the original author and the use of citations when paraphrasing (i.e., summarizing a passage, rearranging the order of a sentence, and changing some of the text; APA, 2010).

Copyright Infringement

The United States Copyright Office defines copyright as "a form of protection grounded in the U.S. Constitution and granted by law for original works of authorship fixed in a tangible medium of expression" (2006, para. 1). Section 106 of the 1976 Copyright Act grants the owner of a copyright the exclusive right to—and to authorize others to—(1) reproduce the work; (2) prepare works derived from the original; (3) distribute copies of the work to the public by sale or other transfer of ownership, or by rental, lease, or lending; (4) perform the work publicly; and (5) display the work publicly (United States Copyright Office, 2012). Works protected by copyright include the following categories: (1) literary, (2) musical, (3) dramatic, (4) pantomime and choreographic, (5) pictorial, graphic, and sculptural, (6) motion pictures and other audiovisual forms, (7) sound recordings, and (8) architectural. The Copyright Office advises viewing the categories broadly, indicating that "computer programs and most 'compilations' may be registered as 'literary works'; maps and architectural plans may be registered as 'pictorial, graphic, and sculptural works'" (United States Copyright Office, 2012, p. 3).

Materials requiring permission, according to the American Psychological Association (APA; 2010), include figures and tables that are reprinted as well as those adapted from or similar to previous works. Although a citation appears to suffice for the use of a table or graphic—after all, a table or graphic is typically a small part of an article—Hough and Priddy (2012) have warned, "A consideration with objects like graphics is that whereas the object itself may be small, it is the percentage of use of that object that is evaluated, not the size of the object. One cannot copy and use an entire graphic because the entire graphic is the entire work" (p. 207). Thus, publishers often require authors to obtain permission to use a table because a table is a work unto itself, and permission is required when using another author's works.

Key for survey scale developers is the APA's (2010) position that permission must be obtained for test and scale items, questionnaires, and vignettes (p. 233). The APA qualified the statement to include especially those items from copyrighted and commercially available tests, such as the Minnesota Multiphasic Personality Inventory and the Stanford-Binet Intelligence Scales. The APA (2010) stated that "a number of commercial instruments—for example, intelligence tests and projective measures—are highly protected. Permission is required, and may be denied, to republish even one item from such instruments" (p. 128). Hough and Priddy (2012) included tests and assessment instruments as being copyright protected.

The APA (2014) muddied the waters by adding, "Obtaining these permissions can be difficult and time-consuming, and a preferable alternative may be to reword or paraphrase those items so as not to duplicate the exact wording" (p. 1). Given the uncertainty of requiring permission to use scale items, we advise if you plan to use items from other instruments, then request permission for those items.

Why be cautious in obtaining permission to use items? Court-ordered compensation for copyright infringement can range from $200 to $150,000 for each infringing copy (Copyright Clearance Center, 2013). In addition, criminal liability is a possibility if one copies a work for financial gain or if the value of the work is more than $1,000.

A request for copyright permission should include print and electronic formats, all future editions, and foreign language editions (APA, 2010). An example of a permission request is shown in Figure 2.3. This request is for a book; however, it could be modified as a request to use materials in an article. For example, the book title would be changed to article title and journal. The information about the tentative price is not relevant and could be deleted. You should keep copies of the permissions in case questions arise (Hough & Priddy, 2012).

Another route for obtaining copyright permission is the Copyright Clearance Center (2013). The Copyright Clearance Center, a nonprofit organization, supports academic institutions in obtaining permission to use and share copyright-protected materials. The Copyright Clearance Center provides copyright services for "millions of in- and out-of-print books, journals, newspapers, magazines, movies, television shows, images, blogs and e-books" (Wikipedia, 2010). Some journals' websites now have a link to the Copyright Clearance Center. To request permission, you click on the permissions tag linked to the article. Once you click the tag, a pop-up window requests information about the material's use (e.g., an article, a book, a dissertation), requestor type (e.g., author, university), format (i.e., print and/or electronic), part (e.g., table, section of the text), and translation (i.e., English and foreign rights).

Adapting or adopting an instrument saves time and resources; however, sometimes the available instruments are outdated or are only tangentially related to the purpose of your study or program evaluation. When a suitable instrument is not available, then developing a survey scale is the next step. Yet, developing your own instrument does not guarantee a sound survey scale. Contributing to the development of a sound instrument are (1) a framework to guide the construction of the scale and (2) guidelines for writing items and developing item response scales. In Chapter 3, we focus on the development of a conceptual framework to guide the development of a survey scale. Subsequently, in Chapters 4 and 5, we provide guidelines for the development of items and their response scales.

Permission Request

I am preparing a manuscript to be published by Guilford Publications, Inc:

Book Title:

Author:

Estimated Publication Date:

Estimated Number of Total Pages:

Approximate Print Run:

Tentative Price:

May I have your permission to use the following material:

Book/Journal title: _____

Author(s) and/or editor(s): _____

Title of Selection: _____

From page _____ to page _____. Copyright Year/Journal Date: _____
_____

Figure # _____ on page _____ Table # _____ on page _____

(If necessary attach continuation sheet or sample of requested material)

in this publication, and in future revisions and editions thereof including non-exclusive world rights in all languages, bookclub rights, electronic rights as that term is commonly understood in the publishing industry, including all rights under U.S. Copyright Law to exploit the Work and derivative works in all electronic and on-line media now known and hereafter to be developed, in all languages throughout the world, including versions made by non-profit organizations for use by blind or physically handicapped persons. It is understood that full credit will be given to the author and publisher.

Please indicate your agreement by signing and returning this form. In signing you warrant that you are the sole owner of the rights granted and that your material does not infringe upon the copyright or other rights of anyone. If you do not control these rights, I would appreciate your letting me know to whom I should apply.

Sincerely,

I (we) grant permission for the use requested above.
_____ Date: _____

Print Name: _____

FIGURE 2.3. Example of a permission request form. Copyright © 2016 The Guilford Press. Reprinted by permission.

FURTHER READING ▨▨▨▨▨▨▨▨▨▨▨

American Psychological Association. (2010). *Publication manual of the American Psychological Association* (6th ed.). Washington, DC: Author.

> *Discusses the issues of copyright permission and plagiarism. Provides guidance for when permission is required.*

Fishman, S. (2011). *The copyright handbook: What every writer needs to know* (11th ed.). Berkeley, CA: Nolo.

> *Presents an in-depth discussion of copyright protection and infringement. Distinguishes between plagiarism and copyright infringement.*

CHAPTER EXERCISES

1. Consider the qualities of reliability and validity. (Refer back to Chapter 1 for a review of these two qualities.) In the section "Reviewing Potential Instruments for Adoption or Adaptation" in this chapter, the step of clarifying instrument purpose will most contribute to the validity of the conclusions we make from the data. How does clarifying the purpose of an instrument contribute to validity?

2. Which step(s) in the "Reviewing Potential Instruments" section will deepen your understanding of other scholars' conceptualization of the construct that is the focus of your data collection?

3. Based on Murray-Ward's review of the Index of Teaching Stress, how would you complete the "Content Evaluation" section of the evaluation guide in Figure 2.1?

4. Reliability ranges from 0 to 1.0. Reliability coefficients from .80 to 1.0 are typically considered to be acceptable. As reported by Murray-Ward, what were the reliability coefficients of the Index of Teaching Stress? Are these acceptable?

5. Considering Murray-Ward's review, if your study focuses on teacher stress, would you adopt, adapt, or reject the Index of Teaching Stress?

6. How does the *Mental Measurements Yearbook* differ from the *Test Collection at ETS*?

7. How does plagiarism differ from copyright infringement?

CHAPTER 3

Establishing a Framework for the Development of a Survey Scale

To some extent everyone already has a conceptual framework,
in that we all have assumptions and presuppositions about how
the world is put together, and we already have a set of concepts
which we use for categorizing things in our experience.
—WILLIAMS (1979, p. 97)

Introduction

The development of a survey scale should be systematic in order to assure the quality of the instrument that will be used to measure the constructs that are the focus of the study. As discussed in Chapter 1, a construct is an attribute or idea expressed in an abstract way. Constructs are instances of concepts that are not directly observable. Examples of constructs include career interests, attitudes toward diversity, and patient satisfaction with health care services. Note that these constructs are not directly observable. This is in contrast to concepts, which include observable phenomena in the form of patterns, categories, or classes of objects. Examples of concepts include forms of poetry, breeds of dogs, types of dairy products, and varieties of sport activities. The focus of *Survey Scales* is the development of survey scales to measure constructs, so in our presentation of conceptual models we refer to "constructs."

Survey scale items are developed to operationalize the construct and its domains (also referred to as components or subscales). The items serve as individual indicators of the underlying construct and its domains. For example, a patient satisfaction construct might be composed of the domains

35

of quality of medical care, interaction with the health care provider, professionalism of clinical staff, and health care facilities. The survey developer operationalizes the construct by writing items relevant to measuring the construct and each of its domains. Once operationalized, a construct can function as a variable in the study of a phenomenon of interest. In our health care example, the variable "interaction with health care provider" might be used to study whether clients' perceptions about the quality of care differ by age.

In this chapter, we examine the use of a conceptual framework to systematize the development of a survey scale. Figures 3.1 and 3.2 provide an example of a model and narrative that together comprise a conceptual framework. You might ask, "How does such a conceptual framework help in developing survey items?" As implied in Williams's statement, a researcher who is faced with myriad constructs (e.g., knowledge, attitudes, and behaviors) related to a research study can develop a conceptual framework to make explicit the constructs that are the focus of the study. These constructs, in turn, guide us in the development of items for a survey scale.

In introducing a study, a conceptual framework includes a narrative in which a researcher articulates the reasons for, and goals of, his or her research (Ravitch & Riggan, 2012). As we discussed in Chapter 1, the narrative defines and describes the constructs in the framework and makes explicit the relationships between the constructs, or variables, in the study.

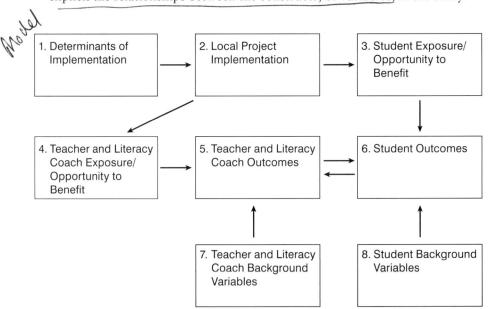

FIGURE 3.1. A model that depicts the constructs and relationships in a conceptual framework that guided an evaluation of a reading intervention.

Narrative

The conceptual framework for Reading First incorporates eight components. The first two components, *Determinants of Implementation* and *Local Project Implementation*, address district and school level variations in program support and program implementation at the local Reading First sites. The *Student Exposure/Opportunity to Benefit, Student Outcomes*, and *Student Background Variables* describe variation among individual students. Similarly, *Teacher and Literacy Coach Exposure/Opportunity to Benefit, Teacher and Literacy Coach Outcomes*, and *Teacher and Literacy Coach Background Variables* deal with variation at the individual level for teachers and literacy coaches. The following sections provide brief overviews of each component and provide illustrative examples of variables that are likely to be included in an assessment of the component. Final specifications of the variables in each component will be determined during the first year of the project following consultation with national and state Reading First Program staff and a review of the documentation provided in local educational agency application materials.

Component 4, *Teacher and Literacy Coach Exposure/Opportunity to Benefit*, provides information on the individual teacher's and literacy coach's experience in the Reading First program and other literacy-related programs. Like students, individual teachers vary in the type and quality of program activities that they experience. Measures for this component are likely to include:

- professional development activities attended at the state, district, and local school level;
- amount of time that the individual teacher or literacy coach has participated in professional development on the essential components of reading instruction, instructional assessment (screening, diagnostic, and classroom), and implementation of scientifically based instructional materials, strategies, and programs;
- opportunities that the teacher has to benefit from interactions with the literacy coach;
- amount of time that coach has spent in university-based professional development; and prior training and participation in literacy-related programs such as the South Carolina Reading Intervention (SCRI), South Carolina READS, Even Start, Head Start, First Steps, etc.

Component 6, *Student Outcomes*, includes the student variables that will provide a meaningful assessment of Reading First impact. The evaluation will examine the effectiveness of Reading First projects in reducing the number of students reading below grade level, as well as the projects' effectiveness in increasing the number of students reading at grade level by low-income, major racial/ethnic groups, limited English proficiency, and special education. In addition, reading scores in Reading First schools will be compared to non-Reading First schools that serve similar student populations and have similar district resources. Variables will include measurement of a student's:

- phonemic awareness
- phonics skills
- fluency
- text comprehension
- vocabulary
- reading level

FIGURE 3.2. Excerpts adapted from the narrative of a conceptual framework that guided the evaluation of a reading intervention. Adapted from the South Carolina Educational Policy Center (2003). Copyright © 2003. Adapted by permission.

The narrative includes the research questions, the hypothesis (i.e., prediction or conjecture about the outcomes of a phenomenon), and the theory that is expressed in the model.

The conceptual model is a diagram that presents the linkages between a set of constructs and their relationships with a phenomenon of interest (Earp & Ennett, 1991; Glatthorn, 1998; Maxwell, 2013; McDavid & Hawthorn, 2006; Miles & Huberman, 1994; Wiersma & Jurs, 2009). Revisit the model (i.e., diagram) in Figure 3.1 and note the linkages between the concepts related to reading literacy. This model of interlinked constructs provides a comprehensive understanding of a phenomenon, in this instance the relationship between teacher development and student achievement. Thus, the term "conceptual framework" refers to the model and narrative that together frame the constructs and relationships that are the focus of one's research study or program evaluation.

Model

Another example of a conceptual model is shown in Figure 3.3. The conceptual model is a diagram or flowchart that uses circles and arrows to depict the proposed links among a set of constructs thought to be related to a specific problem or phenomenon (AERA, 2013; Earp & Ennett, 1991; Glatthorn, 1998; Margoluis & Salafsky, 1998). The model provides a visual representation of the research questions, the constructs that serve as the study variables, and the outcome. The conceptual model in Figure 3.3 guided the development of surveys about the relationships between the behaviors of students, parents, and teachers and the outcome of students' successful transition from middle school to high school. A successful transition was defined as a ninth-grade student being promoted to tenth grade.

The model represents the relation between the **independent variables,** which are thought to influence the outcome, and a **dependent variable,** which is influenced by the independent variables (Margoluis & Salafsky, 1998). In the case of the conceptual model of student transition depicted in Figure 3.3, constructs functioning as the independent variables include grading practices of teachers, school engagement of students, and student–school communication with parents. Of interest to a researcher is whether these independent variables influence the dependent variable (i.e., the promotion of students from ninth grade to tenth grade).

The conceptual framework depicted in Figures 3.1 and 3.2 guided the development of the evaluation questions and data-collection instruments for a reading intervention for elementary students. Accompanying the conceptual model (Figure 3.1) was a narrative (Figure 3.2) that provided brief overviews of each component of the framework and presented variables that could be used to examine the effectiveness of the reading intervention in reducing the number of students reading below grade level.

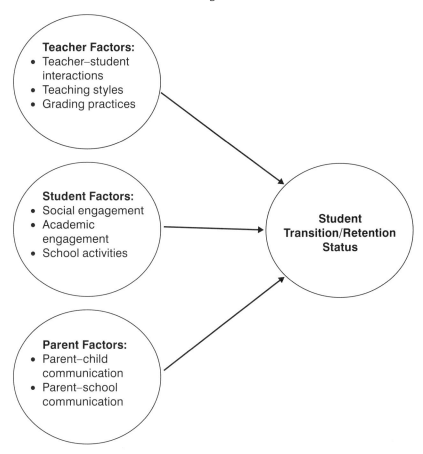

FIGURE 3.3. A conceptual model for the evaluation of a student transition intervention.

Narrative

The conceptual framework requires a narrative to define and describe the constructs (i.e., variables) and make explicit the **propositions** that are implied in the conceptual model. The term *propositions* refers to statements that either (1) define and describe constructs or (2) state the relationship between the constructs in a framework (Fawcett, 1995; Williams, 1979). The statement of the relationship between two or more concepts may take the form of a hypothesis. The relationship examined in Figure 3.1 is whether increased professional development of teachers through their interaction with literacy coaches will be associated with an improvement of student achievement in reading.

Propositions are often stated in vocabulary specific to the field (Fawcett, 1995). For instance, the narrative about the reading intervention (see Figure 3.2) lists specific components of reading: phonemic awareness, phonics skills, fluency, text comprehension, and vocabulary. Although the specific reading skills and strategies associated with these components might be unclear to those outside the field of language and literacy, researchers in the field would understand the components and readily grasp the implications for developing an instrument that gauges, for example, students' phonemic awareness.

Elements and Format

A closer examination of Figures 3.1 and 3.3 shows the elements of a conceptual model. In a conceptual model, circles or boxes represent the constructs that are related to the research study. As mentioned earlier, constructs are instances of concepts that are not directly observable (Colton & Covert, 2007; Hopkins, 1998; Spector, 1992). In Figure 3.3, the variables of social and academic engagement are not directly observable and would be considered constructs.

If constructs are not visible, then how do we gauge their influence on other variables in the model? This is where survey scales prove to be useful. We operationalize a construct by developing survey scales (Colton & Covert, 2007; Wienclaw, 2009). To operationalize a construct, you translate the construct into language that allows you to observe and measure attributes that represent the construct. For example, the construct of social engagement can be assessed in students' responses to survey scale items such as "I have many friends at this school." Students' academic engagement can be gauged using items such as "I read the materials that are being talked about in class."

Labels identify each construct in the conceptual model. The labels should be kept brief and should not contain operational definitions or values of the variables (Earp & Ennett, 1991). Thus, *Social Engagement* would be an appropriate label to use in a conceptual model, whereas the label *Social Engagement: 8 items, 1–4 response scales* would clutter the model and contribute to information overload.

Arrows represent processes and relationships between the constructs (Earp & Ennett, 1991). The direction of the arrows indicates the path of influence. The diagram is generally read from left to right, bottom to top, outside to inside, or cause to outcome (Margoluis & Salafsky, 1998). In Figure 3.3, the path of influence is presented as moving from the independent variables on the left to the dependent variable on the right.

Functions of the Conceptual Framework in the Development of a Survey Scale

Earlier we touched on the purpose of a conceptual framework in the development of a survey scale. We now describe the relationship between conceptual frameworks and survey scales in more depth. In terms of developing an instrument, such as a survey scale, Thorkildsen (2010) advised that validity required investigators to define clear measurement aims. The articulation of a conceptual framework will guide the inquiry and clarify the measurement aims.

A conceptual framework brings a structure that guides the systematic construction of a survey scale and, thus, contributes to the development of an accurate measure of the construct that is being studied. The items in a survey scale are meant to measure an underlying construct. Examples of constructs include job satisfaction, knowledge about cancer, and opinions about the school that a respondent's children attend. However, in survey research, to measure a construct we need to write survey items that operationalize that construct. For example, measuring the construct of job satisfaction might require a researcher to develop items for several subscales: agency management, work schedules, job security, job benefits, and job responsibilities (Morgan, Sherlock, & Ritchie, 2010).

In developing a survey scale, the clear definition of the constructs in a conceptual framework will guide the selection of instruments or the development of survey items (Williams, 1979). Based on the conceptual model in Figure 3.3, survey items need to be developed to operationalize the constructs of social engagement and academic engagement. In terms of academic engagement, items for a survey scale might include:

As a ninth-grade student I . . .

> read the materials that are being talked about in class.
>
> write notes about what I read.
>
> complete my homework assignments.

When developing items for the scale, a framework assists in determining which types of items to include and exclude. The explicit statement of constructs will allow the researcher to determine the fit between survey scale items and those constructs. Items that are off-topic will be deleted, and additional items will be developed when coverage of a construct is sparse.

Another illustration of the fit between the conceptual framework and items in the survey scale is provided in Figure 3.4. The conceptual framework that guided the evaluation of the reading intervention contains

Activities with the Reading First literacy coach	Rarely	Seldom	Sometimes	Often
a. Helping me develop lesson plans	1	2	3	4
b. Helping me with classroom organization	1	2	3	4
c. Modeling lessons	1	2	3	4
d. Team teaching with me	1	2	3	4
e. Observing my teaching	1	2	3	4
f. Providing meaningful feedback about my teaching	1	2	3	4
g. Demonstrating scientifically based reading strategies for instruction	1	2	3	4
h. Developing classroom assessments for reading	1	2	3	4
i. Helping me analyze my student assessment results	1	2	3	4
j. Helping me use student assessment data to improve my teaching	1	2	3	4

FIGURE 3.4. A survey scale with items for the *Teacher and Literacy Coach Exposure/Opportunity to Benefit* component of the conceptual model for the evaluation of a reading intervention. From Office of Program Evaluation/South Carolina Educational Policy Center (2005). Copyright © 2005. Reprinted by permission.

a component labeled *Teacher and Literacy Coach Exposure/Opportunity to Benefit (Component 4)*. A quick read of the survey scale, Reading First Initiative: Classroom Teacher Survey Instrument (Office of Program Evaluation/South Carolina Educational Policy Center, 2005), shows the items address opportunities that the teacher has to benefit from her interactions with the literacy coach in her school. Thus, the conceptual framework guided the development of items for this construct.

Construction of a Conceptual Framework

Recall that a conceptual framework presents an argument for the relevance of (1) a study to the researcher community in a field or (2) an evaluation to the stakeholders in a program. Ravitch and Riggan (2012) wrote that "a conceptual framework should argue convincingly that (1) the research questions are an outgrowth of the argument for relevance; (2) the data to be collected provide the researcher with the raw material to explore the research questions; and (3) the analytic approach allows the researcher to effectively respond to . . . those questions" (p. 7). The following steps provide guidance in developing a conceptual framework.

Review the Literature

The arguments you make about the relevance of a study and its contribution to the field should be informed by a review of the literature. The literature review informs the researcher about the existing theory and research related to the phenomenon of interest (Margoluis & Salafsky, 1998; Maxwell, 2013; Miles & Huberman, 1994). The literature review assists the researcher in identifying constructs that have an important role in influencing the outcome (Glatthorn, 1998). The literature can also provide examples of frameworks and theories from other fields (Williams, 1979).

To identify possible constructs to include in your conceptual framework, in the review of the literature you should identify key terms that you use when discussing the phenomenon (Maxwell, 2013). These terms become the constructs in your framework. Maxwell also suggested selecting one construct and brainstorming to identify related constructs. Subsequently, you retain the constructs most closely related to your research study or program evaluation.

A caution is relevant here. Maxwell (2013) wrote that reliance on reviewing and summarizing a body of theoretical or empirical literature might result in too narrow a focus for a study. In developing a conceptual framework, Maxwell recommended reviewing unpublished papers, dissertations, and grant applications; gaining the insights of advisors with expertise in the field; and drawing on one's experiential knowledge. He also included the use of any pilot study or exploratory research that you conduct as part of the research study.

Construct a Model for the Framework

After reviewing resources related to the phenomenon of interest of your study, draft the diagram that will become your conceptual model. One approach to developing a conceptual model is to begin by identifying the endpoint, that is, the dependent variable or outcome (Earp & Ennett, 1991; Margoluis & Salafsky, 1998). For example, improving student transition (i.e., increasing the percentage of ninth-grade students being promoted to tenth grade) is the endpoint in Figure 3.3. The improvement of student achievement in reading and language is the desired outcome in Figure 3.1.

On identification of the outcome, then identify possible independent variables and the initial relationships among the concepts (Earp & Ennett, 1991). Next, narrow the set of variables to those that can be addressed in the research study. The model should not incorporate all variables associated with the endpoint; rather the model will represent a small part of the web associated with a research study (Earp & Ennett, 1991; Fawcett, 1995; Greca & Moreira, 2000; Margoluis & Salafsky, 1998; Maxwell, 2013). For example, the conceptual model about student transition could have included additional variables, such as peer influence; however, collecting data about such a factor was beyond the scope of the study.

Once you identify the relevant variables for your study, use arrows to draw linkages among the constructs (Margoluis & Salafsky, 1998). Paths of influence can be depicted by an arrow that originates from an independent variable and points to the dependent variable. As shown in Figure 3.3, in one format the outcome variable is placed on the right of the diagram and to the left are the independent variables that might influence the outcome.

You should aim to limit the model to a single page; this will allow you to grasp the totality of the phenomenon and the relationship between the constructs (Miles & Huberman, 1994; Robson, 1993). The model should be well organized and relatively simple. A conceptual model presents a simplified reality and includes only the information relevant to the researcher.

Your conceptual model will benefit from your drafting several versions of the visual representations of the concepts and their relationships (Glatthorn, 1998). Subsequently, you select the version of the diagram that best represents the constructs and relationships associated with a phenomenon.

Write the Narrative for the Framework

As you develop your conceptual framework, begin writing the narrative that describes the elements of the framework (Glatthorn, 1998; Margoluis & Salafsky, 1998; Maxwell, 2013). Include in the narrative your initial draft of the research questions, the hypotheses, and the theory that is expressed in the model. The narrative should provide the definitions of the constructs and describe the data to be collected. In preparing to write about the constructs (i.e., the boxes or circles) and processes (i.e., the arrows), ask yourself how the constructs are related and explain the meaning of each arrow (Maxwell, 2013). You will also want to discuss the analyses to be conducted. The narrative will benefit from your drafting multiple versions in tandem with the conceptual model.

Refine the Framework

After developing an initial version of the framework, the next step is to refine it. To do so, share it with stakeholders and other researchers in the field (Margoluis & Salafsky, 1998; Williams, 1979). Options for obtaining feedback include interviewing stakeholders or conducting a focus group with knowledgeable stakeholders.

Although conceptual frameworks are frequently associated with qualitative methodology (e.g., Maxwell, 2013; Miles & Huberman, 1994), Ravitch and Riggan (2012) argued that "the development of conceptual frameworks is a critical process for researchers using qualitative, quantitative, and mixed methods approaches" (p. 152). We concur with Ravitch and Riggan about the important role of a conceptual framework in the research process. Use of the conceptual framework for your research design to guide the development of items will provide validity evidence about your survey scales. Thus, use of the conceptual framework for your research design to inform item development appears critical. In Chapter 4, we discuss the development of survey scale items.

FURTHER READING

Earp, J., & Ennett, S. (1991). Conceptual models for health education research and practice. *Health Education Research: Theory and Practice, 6*(2), 163–171.

> *Provides a thorough discussion of the development of a conceptual framework. Offers numerous examples of conceptual models.*

Maxwell, J. (2013). *Qualitative research design: An interactive approach* (3rd ed.). Thousand Oaks, CA: Sage.

> *Dedicates a chapter to the development of a conceptual model. Uses many examples.*

CHAPTER EXERCISES

1. In Figure 3.1, student attitudes could be a variable for which component?

2. In a job satisfaction survey, the subscales Supervisory Relationship and Job Environment are examples of what elements of a conceptual framework?

3. Consider independent and dependent variables. Provide an example of an independent variable that influences a dependent variable.

4. How does a conceptual framework contribute to the development of a survey scale?

CHAPTER 4

Item-Writing Guidelines

*The words used in a question will always influence
how study participants answer that question.*
—PETERSON (2000, p. 46)

Introduction

Peterson's statement reminds us of the critical choices we make in writing survey items. Given that the words in a survey item will influence the response of a study participant, we want to take care to write items in a way that the responses will allow us to make valid inferences (e.g., decisions, predictions) about the study participants. In Chapter 4, we present guidelines that will help survey developers to write items that are clear to the respondents and that will assess the construct of interest and its domains. Dimensions to guide item writing include (1) relevance to the survey purpose and construct, (2) audience, (3) language, (4) item structure, and (5) conventions.

Addressing Relevance

Relevance is the degree to which an item aligns with the construct and domains that are the focus of the survey scale. The following guidelines will assist you in writing items that support relevance and limit the introduction of error into your survey results.

The Construct of Interest

Relevance requires that an item measures the concept or construct that is the focus of the survey scale (see Table 4.1). Before you begin writing items, you should make explicit the construct and its domains that you want to measure with the survey scale. Specifying the construct and its domains supports the item writer in determining whether an item is related to the survey purpose (DeVellis, 2012).

Return to the conceptual framework in Figure 3.3 and the depiction of the constructs related to student transition/retention status (i.e., passing or failing). In this instance, relevant construct domains include social engagement and academic engagement. This listing reminds us of the construct domains that we should include in the survey and prevents us from including irrelevant items.

Review the item in Figure 4.1 to consider whether it should be included in a student engagement scale. If the domain of interest in Figure 4.1 is student *social* engagement in the high school setting, a question arises about the appropriateness of the item "As a ninth-grade student I know my way around the school." In a social engagement scale, the purpose is to assess the student's connection to other students and his or her teachers. Thus, this item might be deleted from the pool of survey items related to the domain of social engagement. Does the alternative item—"As a ninth-grade student I have many friends at school"—address the domain of social engagement? If so, then it is a candidate for the engagement scale.

Logically Related to the Construct

In beginning to write items, think creatively about the construct and its domains (DeVellis, 2012). Ask yourself, "What are alternative ways that I can word an item to measure the construct?" This process will be facilitated

---

TABLE 4.1. Guidelines for Addressing Relevance

- Develop items that address the construct of interest.
- Write items that are logically related to the survey purpose.
- Use multiple items to tap into a construct, but avoid repetition of items.
- Avoid items that crossover to a related construct (e.g., social anxiety rather than test anxiety).
- Write items to be concrete and precise.
- Keep items and words within an item relevant.
- Keep items objective.

	NOT THIS			
7. As a ninth-grade student I . . .	Strongly disagree	Disagree	Agree	Strongly agree
a. know my way around the school.	1	2	3	4
	BUT THIS			
7. As a ninth-grade student I . . .	Strongly disagree	Disagree	Agree	Strongly agree
a. have many friends at school.	1	2	3	4

FIGURE 4.1. Revisions to items to support relevance.

if your writing is grounded in a review of the literature and examination of similar scales.

As part of the creative generation of items, return to the items that you draft and examine their relevance in gauging the construct of interest. This review will safeguard against the inclusion of items that are not logically related to the survey purpose. Reviewing the conceptual model helps to ensure that items are logically related to the construct domains. Consider, for example, writing items to assess factors related to successful student transition from eighth to ninth grade. At first glance, the statement "My teacher gives checklists or rubrics to us as we prepare to do projects" appears unrelated to the topic. However, if the conceptual model includes a teacher factor as a potential contributor to student transition (see Figure 3.3), then writing items for a subscale that measures teacher assessment practices is appropriate.

Multiple Items

In developing items for a scale, it is generally good practice to write multiple items that measure each domain of the construct that the survey scale measures. Writing multiple items for inclusion in a survey scale supports the researcher in better assessing the breadth of the construct and supporting the consistency of domain scores.

Multiple Items for Consistency

Typically, a score from a construct domain is composed of several items. For example, a classroom climate subscale might include multiple items that measure teacher instructional practices:

My teacher checks to see if we are understanding the classwork.

My teacher makes it easy for me to ask questions.

My teacher tells us what to study to prepare for a test.

(adapted from Johnson, Davis, Fisher, Johnson, & Somerindyke, 2000)

Using several items to form a score for the domain of classroom climate will support score consistency more than using a single item. Consistency of scores is related to the reliability of scores, a topic we explore in depth in Chapter 8.

The need for multiple items, however, is not addressed by repeating an item after minor changes to that item. Respondents might perceive repetitive items as irrelevant (Peterson, 2000). Consider the following item from a scale on classroom climate: "My teachers respect me." Students might perceive as irrelevant a repetitious item that states, "I am respected by my teachers." An item that taps into respect, but is not simply a repetition of another item, is "My teachers care about what I have to say."

Multiple Items for Content Representativeness

Multiple items also are needed to measure a construct that is composed of several domains. Multiple items specific to each domain will ensure that the items are representative of the construct and its domains. In the Caregiver Survey (see Morgan et al., 2010: see Table 1.2), the scale has three domains: job satisfaction, supervisory relationships, and job environment. Thus, items had to be developed for all three domains. Examples of potential items that address a job environment domain include:

I am involved in challenging work.

I have a chance to gain new skills on the job.

Items for the supervisory relationship domain might include

My supervisor is open to new ideas.

My supervisor is available to answer questions when I need help with my clients.

My supervisor tells me when I am doing a good job.

My supervisor is responsive with problems that affect my job.

(adapted from Morgan et al., 2010)

Notice that the two domains of supervisory relationships and job environment represent two different, but related, expressions of a complex condition or phenomenon, that is, job satisfaction. Thus, we need multiple items for purposes of consistency and for adequate assessment of the breadth of the construct.

Crossover

Relevance also requires avoiding items that cross over to a related construct. Such a crossover is evident in the item "As a ninth-grade student I care if I finish high school." This statement appears to measure a generalized engagement (or disengagement) of the student rather than academic or social engagement.

Concrete and Precise

Writing items that are concrete and precise will avoid ambiguity. Items gauging teachers' attitudes about inclusion of students with special needs in the classroom illustrate the need for items to be unambiguous. Contrast the following statements related to inclusion of students with disabilities in a general education classroom:

> Inclusion is good for all children.
>
> Inclusion is good for most children.
>
> (Stanley, n.d.)

Does a high score on inclusion being good for *all* children translate to a high score for the construct of teacher's attitude toward inclusion? Then does a high score on inclusion being good for *most* children translate to a high score for the construct of teacher's attitude toward inclusion? Does a teacher indicating that inclusion is good for *most* children translate to a low score for the construct? Thus, the items are ambiguous in terms of a teacher's attitude toward inclusion.

Item and Word Relevance

Survey scale items must be relevant, and the words that constitute an item must be relevant. Consider using the item "As a ninth-grade student I come to school only because my friends are here." The intent of the item appears appropriate—to gauge the importance of a student's friends in motivating him or her to come to school. However, the term "only" muddies the meaning. If the student strongly agrees, then is that response—"I strongly agree that I come to school *only* because my friends are here"—positive in terms of social engagement in a school setting? If the item is revised to say that "I come to school to see my friends," then the focus of the item appears to more closely gauge the construct of social engagement in the school setting.

Objectivity

Relevance also requires the survey developer to maintain objectivity in items. Nonobjective items suggest the correct answer; such leading items discredit the researcher. A nonobjective item uses emotionally laden language that will introduce bias and interfere with the interpretation of respondents' answers. One will not know if responses reflect study participants' reaction to the biased language or to the content of the items. The following item is from the Research Committee of the Sierra Club (n.d.):

> Our nation is still blessed with millions of acres of public lands, including roadless wilderness areas, forests and range lands. Land developers, loggers, and mining and oil companies want to increase their operations on these public lands. *Do you think these remaining pristine areas of your public lands should be protected from such exploitation?*
>
> ☐ Yes   ☐ No   ☐ No Opinion

The emotionally charged language in this item makes clear the answer desired by the surveyors. The bias in the item is likely to call into question the credibility of the research committee conducting the survey.

Addressing Audience

A major consideration in writing items is that of audience (see Table 4.2). In considering audience, we ask, "What are the characteristics of the survey respondents?"

Cognitive Skills and Communication

As you write items, you should take into account the cognitive skills and communication capabilities of the survey respondents. For example, will respondents be children or adults? Is the language that you use in your items

TABLE 4.2. Guidelines for Audience
• Consider the cognitive skills and communication capabilities of the respondents and their ability to understand an item.
• Determine if respondents will have sufficient information to answer the items.
• Consider if the study participants will be able to recall the information (e.g., behaviors, activities).
• Represent the diversity of respondents (i.e., multicultural, nonbias).

appropriate for the age group? For high school students, you might use the following statement, "Participation in the *Discovery Workshop* improved my written communication skills." However, for elementary students you might say, "Being in the *Discovery Workshop* improved my writing." The reading level is demanding for both items; however, the reading level for the latter statement for the elementary students is less demanding than the item written for high school students.

Sufficient Information

Determining whether respondents will have sufficient information to answer items will contribute to the development of appropriate items. Ask yourself, "Will respondents have sufficient knowledge to answer this item?" This guideline addresses the ability of the respondent to provide the desired information. We distinguish this guideline from the respondent's understanding of the topic (i.e., knowledge), which is addressed later in this chapter. Figure 4.2 provides an illustration of an item that asks students how frequently their teacher meets with students who are having difficulty with their work. In deciding whether this item should be used in a student survey, you should ask yourself whether students are likely to know if a teacher assists *other* students before or after school. Do not expect accurate answers when asking respondents what others do or feel (Nardi, 2003).

A second issue is whether the students are likely to know how frequently a teacher meets with students who need assistance. Although a student might know that her teacher has a policy of assisting students during lunch, the student is unlikely to know the frequency with which other students receive assistance from the teacher during lunch.

Recall of Information

Respondents' ability to recall information about activities and behaviors should also be considered. In gauging respondents' ability to recall information, use a time period related to the importance of the item topic. Peterson

4. My English teacher . . .	Rarely	Sometimes	Often	Frequently
f. meets during lunch with students who are having difficulty with their work.	1	2	3	4

FIGURE 4.2. Example of an item that asks for information that is unavailable to the respondent.

(2000) warned against asking respondents about practices over a long time period and recommended focusing on a short time period for which the respondent is likely to recall events or daily practices. Important information, such as major life events, can be recalled over a longer time period, whereas commonplace events might be recalled for only the previous few weeks or months (Fink, 2003; Fowler, 1995).

Representation of Diversity

Attention to diversity is another aspect of audience. In developing items, the writer should consider the diversity of the survey respondents and ensure the various groups would perceive the survey as relevant. For example, retirees might consider irrelevant any items that ask about behaviors in the office setting. The relevance of the language used in the items should also be reviewed by members of the various groups that will be completing the survey scale. This review can be achieved by conducting focus groups with participants similar to those who will complete the **operational** survey.

The issue of audience cannot be separated from language, conventions, and item structure. Thus, as you develop items, you should revisit the issue of audience to inform decisions related to these qualities of surveys.

Addressing Language

In the writing of an item, attention should be paid to the language in order to craft items that the study participants will understand. Contrast presenting parents with the stimulus "I visit the school for educational functions" versus the statement "I attend school events." Some parents might be confused by the term "functions" but understand the word "events." This example shows the importance of attending to word choice and the demands of language in writing an item.

Language Understood by Respondents

The first guideline in Table 4.3 advises using language that will be understood by the study participants. The item in Figure 4.3 uses straightforward language—*makes it easy for me to ask questions* rather than *facilitates asking questions*. In using the term *me*, the item developer expresses the item in the context of the student's experience.

Respondents must be familiar with the vocabulary used in the items. Study participants might respond to items with unfamiliar vocabulary; however, their responses might be inconsistent owing to their partial understanding of the item. Recall that the intent of the researcher is to make inferences/draw conclusions about the participants' attitudes, knowledge,

TABLE 4.3. Guidelines for Addressing Language (Vocabulary)

- Use words with meanings understood by respondents.
- Use language (i.e., terms, concepts) that is current.
- Avoid words with multiple meanings.
- Attend to word choices.
- Avoid abstractions.
- Write items at middle school level reading demands for the general public.

or behaviors. A researcher might arrive at inappropriate conclusions if the language demands of survey items result in responses counter to the intent of study participants. For example, in a school climate survey, some parents might correctly interpret the phrase "students retained" to mean the percentage of students who were not promoted to the next grade level, whereas other parents might interpret the phrase as providing information about the graduation rate. Respondents' interpretation of a statistic, for example, 6.2%, is likely to be very different if parents think the statistic reflects the percentage of students who must repeat a grade versus the percentage of students who graduate. Although parents who initially interpret the information as being related to graduation will likely self-correct, in developing a survey scale we want to write items that are clear in their intent.

Items with numerous technical terms might result in respondents appearing to have little knowledge about a topic; however, if the items had been presented in lay terms, then the survey respondents could have demonstrated their understanding. In Figure 4.4, the item could be edited to delete the term "transition" and make the item more understandable to students.

⊘ NOT THIS				
3. My teacher . . .	**Rarely**	**Sometimes**	**Often**	**Frequently**
e. facilitates asking questions.	1	2	3	4
✓ BUT THIS				
3. My teacher . . .	**Rarely**	**Sometimes**	**Often**	**Frequently**
e. makes it easy for me to ask questions.	1	2	3	4

FIGURE 4.3. Example of an item that uses the language of the respondent.

Based on your opinion about how well you are doing in school, indicate how well the following aspects of the Quest Center prepared you for middle school.

🚫 NOT THIS

a. The math round tables at the Quest Center prepared me for transition to middle school mathematics.	1 Strongly disagree	2 Disagree	3 Agree	4 Strongly agree

✓ BUT THIS

a. The math round tables at the Quest Center prepared me for mathematics in middle school.	1 Strongly disagree	2 Disagree	3 Agree	4 Strongly agree

FIGURE 4.4. Example of an item with demanding vocabulary.

Current Language

Another consideration in writing items is to use language that is current. For example, in special education, one no longer refers to a learning-disabled child; rather, one speaks of a child with a learning disability (University of Kansas Research and Training Center on Independent Living, 2008). Instead of using the term "homosexual," one should use "gay men" or "lesbians" (APA, 2010). Notice that the language here also overlaps with the issue of diversity discussed previously.

Multiple-Meaning Words

Words with multiple meanings have the potential to create confusion, so they should be avoided. The phrase "school environment information," for example, has multiple meanings. Does the researcher want information about the physical environment, such as air quality, structural integrity, or handicap accessibility? Or do researchers want information about teacher and student morale, parental involvement, and school safety? If multiple-meaning words cannot be avoided, then the context of the item should clearly establish the meaning of the word within the item.

Choices about Words

To improve respondent understanding of survey items, one should attend to word choices and select wording that is meaningful to study participants. So, when writing, avoid highly technical words, infrequently used words, slang, colloquialisms, jargon, and abbreviations. You should also avoid words with multiple syllables. As with any guideline, there will be exceptions to the rule. For example, the technical language associated with a field, such as public health, might appear to be jargon for those outside of the field but convey the appropriate meaning to public health educators. For instance, although the term "body mass index" and its related acronym, BMI, are commonplace in the public health field, for those outside the field the language might be unfamiliar.

Abstractions

In selecting wording, you should avoid abstractions. For example, do not ask about behavior in terms of "average." Asking a respondent the number of books that he or she reads on average each month is a cognitively demanding task. It is better to ask the typical number of books a respondent reads each month. In Figure 4.5, the phrase "climate for implementation" is an abstraction. What is a climate for implementation? Does this have to do with principal support? Is it in reference to professional training having been completed to prepare teachers for implementation of a magnet program? Is the term addressing parent support of a magnet? If it is the latter, then the item could be written as "Parents are supportive of the magnet program."

Reading Demands

For the general public, the reading demands of a survey should be at the fifth- to eighth-grade level (Barnette, 2010; Peterson, 2000). The spelling and grammar tool in Microsoft Word provides an estimate of the reading level for a document (Microsoft Corporation, 2010). To obtain an estimate for an item or a document, highlight the text for which you want to estimate a reading level, click the Review tab, and click the Spelling & Grammar option. A pop-up window states that Word has completed checking the selection and asks whether you want it to check the rest of the document. When you select No, another pop-up with the readability indices appears.[1]

Two useful indices of reading levels are the Flesch–Kincaid Grade Level and the Flesch Reading Ease (Microsoft Corporation, 2010). In Figure 4.5, the top item on a positive school climate has a Flesch–Kincaid Grade Level index of 9.4, which means a ninth-grade student should understand the text. In contrast, the bottom item on supportive parents in Figure 4.5 has a Flesch–Kincaid Grade Level index of 7.3 (seventh grade, third month), indicating the revised item is slightly easier to read.

---

[1]In Word 2013, if a pop-up window does not appear with the readability statistics, then go to REVIEW → LANGUAGE → LANGUAGE PREFERENCES → PROOFING and check the "show readability statistics" option.

NOT THIS						
	Strongly disagree	Disagree	Slightly disagree	Slightly agree	Agree	Strongly agree
23. The climate for implementation of the magnet program is positive in my school.	O	O	O	O	O	O

BUT THIS						
	Strongly disagree	Disagree	Slightly disagree	Slightly agree	Agree	Strongly agree
23. Parents are supportive of the magnet program.	O	O	O	O	O	O

FIGURE 4.5. Example of an item with an abstraction.

The Flesch Reading Ease has a 100-point scale. As the score increases, the document is easier to read. With a score of 54.7, the item about parent support in Figure 4.5 is fairly easy to read. The scores for both readability indices are based on the average number of syllables per word and the number of words per sentence (Microsoft Corporation, 2010). Thus, you can control the reading level required by your assessments by avoiding words with multiple syllables and by attending to the length of the sentences.

Addressing Item Structure

The complexity of an item can be controlled by following the guidelines in Table 4.4. Items should be as brief as possible and still clearly communicate to the survey respondent what the researcher is asking.

Brevity

Peterson (2000) recommended keeping items brief. To achieve brevity, he recommended limiting an item to 20 words or less and using no more than three commas. In a survey, each word is associated with a cost, such as the direct cost of web development and the indirect cost of a respondent's time. Adherence to the guideline of brevity helps to control these costs. Recall also that reading level is, in part, a function of sentence length and brevity will reduce reading demands.

TABLE 4.4. Guidelines for Addressing Item Structure

- Write items to be brief.

- Write complete statements.

- Present a single idea in an item.

- Use positive wording instead of negative phrasing.

- Begin items with qualifying clauses because respondents begin to formulate a response before the item is complete.

- Reduce the reading load by eliminating repetition in the phrasing of items.

Complete Sentences

To keep items short and simple, you might be tempted to use phrases for some items. For example, in the demographics section of a survey you might be tempted to use the following:

Year of birth?

Survey developers, however, warn against such a shortcut. Using phrases instead of complete statements likely increases the cognitive demands for the respondent. In essence, the survey respondent must fill in the gaps and mentally "write" the item to read, "What is your year of birth?" Thus, to keep the demands of the survey low for the respondents, items should be written as complete statements, not as phrases.

Single Idea

The complexity of an item is reduced, and the interpretability increases, when a statement or question focuses only on one idea. As shown in Figure 4.6, the survey respondents are asked whether their English teachers write comments about the strengths and weaknesses of the students' graded work. This item fails to focus on one idea. Is a student to respond in regards to his or her teacher's written comments about weaknesses or to the teacher's comments about strengths? Some teachers mark weaknesses; so perhaps the student should circle *Often* or *Almost all the time*. But what if the teacher rarely writes comments about students' strengths? If the items were written to focus on one idea, then the task is straightforward. One way to guard against items with more than one focus is to watch for use of the word "and" in an item. Often the term "and" is used to join two ideas in an item and serves as a cue that the ideas should be split into two items.

4. My English teacher . . .	Rarely	Sometimes	Often	Almost all the time
f. writes comments about the strengths and weaknesses of my graded work.	1	2	3	4

NOT THIS (above)

BUT THIS (below)

4. My English teacher . . .	Rarely	Sometimes	Often	Almost all the time
f. writes comments about the *strengths* of my graded work.	1	2	3	4
g. writes comments about the *weaknesses* of my graded work.	1	2	3	4

FIGURE 4.6. Example of an item that focuses on a single idea.

An item that gauges teachers' attitudes toward inclusion provides another illustration of the need for an item to have a single focus. Classroom teachers were asked to respond to the following item, "Working with the consultant teacher takes valuable time away from planning and student time." If a teacher strongly agrees with the statement, then is the problem with planning time, student time, or both?

The presentation of a single idea is critical in the use of true–false items. Examine the following item. This item asks about alcohol *and* smoking.

5. Women who smoke and drink more than one alcoholic beverage a day increase their risk for breast cancer.

(adapted from University of Rochester Medical Center, 2014)

If a survey respondent answers this item correctly, is it because he knew that both smoking and alcohol were risks associated with breast cancer? Or did the participant answer it correctly because he knew smoking increased the risk but he was less certain about alcohol consumption?

Positive Wording

Using positive wording instead of negative phrasing also reduces the complexity of an item. For example, a survey respondent must perform mental gymnastics to answer the item "The budget for teacher resources at the Quest Center is *not* adequate." A respondent might ask herself, "If I mark strongly disagree, then I think the budget is adequate, right? If I mark strongly agree, then the budget is not adequate?" That the item requires the respondent to decode its meaning is problematic. Faced with multiple items that are cognitively demanding, the respondent might not complete the survey.

Qualifying Phrases

Qualifying clauses should occur at the beginning of a survey item because respondents begin to formulate a response before the item is complete (Peterson, 2000). So, if an item states, "I really feel that I am a member of a team within the FAME magnet program," then a teacher might formulate his response based on his sense of belonging to the school in general (i.e., "I really feel that I am a member of a team"). To gauge the teacher's sense of belonging to the magnet program, the item should be phrased, "Within the FAME magnet program, I really feel that I am a member of a team."

Eliminating Repetitive Phrasing

Items within a scale often begin with similar phrasing. In Figure 4.7, each item begins with the phrasing "Consultation on. . . . " The reading demands of the item can be reduced by creating a stem with the repeated words. Note the ease in determining the focus of each item when the repetitive material is removed.

Addressing Conventions

Attending to conventions helps to create a professional look for a survey. A survey that fails to follow conventions and is riddled with typographical errors sends the wrong message to survey respondents about their value. The guidelines offered in this section provide reminders about creating a survey that conveys to survey respondents their importance to a study.

Language Conventions

In writing items, Peterson (2000) advised following standard language conventions, such as avoiding double negatives in items. As shown in Table 4.5, the items in the survey scale should be reviewed to ensure the items follow standard language conventions, including spelling, punctuation, and

	Strongly dissatisfied	Dissatisfied	Satisfied	Strongly satisfied
⊘ NOT THIS				
Satisfaction with Communication Center Services for Students				
Consultation on resume writing	1	2	3	4
Consultation on academic assignments	1	2	3	4
Consultation on business writing	1	2	3	4
Consultation on thesis/dissertation	1	2	3	4
✓ BUT THIS				
Satisfaction with Communication Center Services for Students				
Consultation on . . .				
academic assignments	1	2	3	4
business writing	1	2	3	4
resume writing	1	2	3	4
thesis/dissertation	1	2	3	4

FIGURE 4.7. Example of reducing the reading load of an item.

grammar. Attention to conventions will reduce the likelihood that errors will interfere with survey participants' understanding and their responses.

Typographical Errors

As the drafting of items comes to a close, you need to review the items for typographical errors. Microsoft Word uses red underlining to show potential spelling errors or green underlining to indicate possible grammatical

---

TABLE 4.5. Guidelines for Addressing Language Conventions

- Follow standard language conventions.
- Review for typographical errors.

issues. However, in developing items and attending to all the guidelines that we have discussed, it is easy to overlook markings and not correct typographical errors. That is, sometimes in our haste to complete the development of a survey, we forget to page through the document for errors. Also, sometimes incorrectly used terms are not flagged by a word-processing application because they are correctly spelled, but they are not the intended words. For example, if I misspelled "words" as "works," a word-processing program might not flag it because it is a correctly spelled word.

A survey with typographical errors might create confusion for the respondents. Also, typographical errors might raise questions about the researcher's credibility. Surveys that have been edited for conventions and typographical errors express a sense of professionalism and convey to respondents the importance of their role in the research effort.

Guidelines Specific to Item Type

In the following section, we present guidelines specific to item type: knowledge, behavior, and demographics.

Guidelines Specific to Knowledge-Based Items

In Chapter 1, we raised the possibility of using true–false item formats to gauge survey respondents' knowledge of a topic. The item-writing guidelines in the previous sections of this chapter apply to developing knowledge-based, true–false items. That is, in writing true–false items, one must be sure that the items align with the construct that is the focus of the survey scale. The audience must be considered; the language written must be clear and at the appropriate reading level for the survey respondents; and items written need to be brief and to clearly communicate the intent of the items and the conventions of language followed. Although there is considerable overlap in guidelines for item writing, the true–false format has some issues specific to that type of item. Guidelines specific to writing true–false items are listed in Table 4.6.

TABLE 4.6. Guidelines Specific to Knowledge Items

- Do not mix partly true with partly false statements.
- Avoid a disproportionate number of correct true and correct false responses.
- Avoid specific determiners (e.g., "all," "none").
- Consider the use of variants of the true–false form.

Partly True–Partly False

In the use of true–false items, do not mix partially true with partially false statements. If we want clarity in an item, then the statement must be either true or false, not both. Consider the following statement:

> 3. A healthy diet includes plenty of whole grains, fruits, vegetables, and saturated fat.
>
> (adapted from University of Arkansas for Medical Sciences, 2014)

A healthy diet does include plenty of whole grains, fruits, and vegetables, so the statement appears true. However, plenty of saturated fat is not part of a healthy diet, so is the statement false? We do not want to require survey respondents to internally debate the intent of the true–false statement. Better to use two items:

> A healthy diet includes plenty of whole grains, fruits, and vegetables.
>
> Saturated fat is part of a balanced diet.

Balancing True–False Statements

Should you use mainly true statements, more false than true items, or equal amounts of both? Early researchers advised using more false items because when respondents are uncertain of an answer, they are likely to guess the answer is true (Cronbach, 1946, 1950; Gustav, 1963). Ebel (1965) suggested that 60% of items should be false.

Specific Determiners

Specific determiners, such as "all," "always," and "never," cue the respondent that a statement is likely false. In contrast, modifiers such as "generally," "sometimes," and "many" provide a clue that a statement is true. Hopkins (1998) suggested that balancing the number of true and false items that use specific determiners can decrease the influence of such modifiers on respondents' answers.

Variants of the True–False Form

A variation of the true–false format involves using an item format with alternate choices. Figure 4.8 shows two items that provide alternate choices for respondents to select. Each item presents a brief scenario that describes classroom assessment practices that are ethical or unethical (Johnson, Green, Kim, & Pope, 2008).

---

1. A teacher assesses student knowledge by using many types of assessments: multiple-choice tests, essays, projects, portfolios.

   O Ethical

   O Unethical

16. A teacher allows a student with a learning disability in language arts to use a tape-recorder when the student answers the essay questions on social studies tests.

   O Ethical

   O Unethical

FIGURE 4.8. Alternate choice items for assessing educators' understanding of ethical classroom assessment practices.

Study participants (preservice teachers, teachers, and administrators) marked whether each assessment practice was ethical or unethical. Based on the literature on assessment, Johnson et al. (2008) developed an answer guide and scored participants' responses as correct or incorrect. These scores provided information about the survey participants' understanding of ethical practices. To the degree that respondents' selection of myth/fact and ethical/unethical scenarios are similar to the selection of true and false items, more myth items and more unethical items appear appropriate (see the earlier section "Balancing True–False Statements").

Related to the true–false format is the checklist format. The items shown in Figure 4.9 can serve to gauge teachers' understanding of the types of assessments that are appropriate for assessing students' progress in reading. The scoring of teachers' responses would be guided by the researcher's theoretical framework of reading. For example, whole language focuses on how students make sense of the text as they read (Taylor, 2007). Teaching and assessment within this framework is characterized by the principle of authenticity of texts, tasks, and tests and integration of reading, writing, speaking, and listening (Pearson, 2004). Within this framework, if a teacher checks portfolios as one appropriate method for monitoring student reading progress, then the researcher can count the response correct if portfolios provide information about how students make meaning of text as they read. In contrast, if a teacher checks end-of-chapter core reading tests (i.e., multiple-choice tests), then the researcher might consider the response incorrect because such tests often rely on reading passages that are written for the sole purpose of testing reading skills and do not engage students in authentic reading experiences. Thus, the researcher would review each classroom assessment, use the theoretical framework to determine if each

Please indicate which of the following classroom assessments are appropriate for monitoring students' reading progress. **Please select all that apply**.

____ Anecdotal notes

____ Conferencing with students

____ Core reading tests (supplied by publisher)

____ Miscue analysis

____ Observation

____ Running records

____ Spelling tests

____ Student portfolios

____ Teacher-made tests (e.g., multiple choice, short answer, matching)

____ Vocabulary tests

____ Worksheets

____ Writing samples

____ Other (Please specify in box below)

FIGURE 4.9. Checklist to gauge teachers' understanding of appropriate assessment practices.

assessment practice was appropriate, develop a key for scoring teachers' responses, and score and tally each teacher's correct responses.

Assessing Knowledge versus Perceptions about Knowledge

The intent of the previous examples is to test respondents to measure their understanding of important knowledge. In some instances, the researcher might develop a survey scale in which respondents self-report *perceptions* about their knowledge level. The items in Figure 4.10 do not actually "test" a respondent to measure his or her knowledge about a topic; rather, the items ask for the respondent's perceptions about his or her understanding of technology.

Guidelines for Items about Behaviors

A survey scale also might address behaviors (e.g., walking, jogging, golf, basketball; Peterson, 2000). When measuring behaviors, items are often accompanied by a frequency response scale, which will be discussed in more detail in Chapter 5. If one wants to measure parent involvement in their

I know how to . . .		Yes	No
a.	turn the desktop on and off.	O	O
b.	log onto the network.	O	O
c.	conduct research on the Internet.	O	O
d.	use Microsoft Word.	O	O
e.	use Microsoft Publisher.	O	O
f.	use Microsoft PowerPoint.	O	O
g.	use Microsoft Excel.	O	O
h.	use CPS clickers.	O	O
i.	use SMARTBoard (write on it, erase, and move objects).	O	O

FIGURE 4.10. Example of an item that assesses student *perceptions* about knowledge.

child's school, then the survey scale might include the item in Figure 4.11. Note that the response scale is a frequency scale ("Rarely"–"Frequently") and not a satisfaction scale (i.e., "Dissatisfied"–"Satisfied").

Parent involvement could also be measured by using a checklist of behaviors as shown in Figure 4.12. Contrast the Likert-style item in Figure 4.11 with the checklist-formatted item in Figure 4.12. The major difference is that the checklist captures the different types of activities parents might engage in but not the frequency of the behaviors. The list of behaviors could be developed through reviewing the literature and conducting a focus group with some parents, perhaps the members of a school improvement committee or the Parent, Teacher, Student Association.

To ensure that all respondents consider the same timeframe, you should specify the time period for which they report their activities. Recall that earlier we discussed the Peterson's recommendation (2000) to avoid asking respondents about practices over a long time period if respondents will be asked to recall events or daily practices. However, Fink (1995) warned to avoid too short a time period because less frequently occurring events may

Academic Year 2017	Rarely	Sometimes	Often	Frequently
I attended school events.	1	2	3	4

FIGURE 4.11. Example of an item to measure parents' involvement in their children's school.

22. Please check all the volunteer activities in which you participated at the Center for the Arts during the 2016–2017 school year.

____ act as a homeroom parent

____ accompany students on field trips

____ listen to students read

____ participate as a classroom volunteer

____ read to students

____ serve on the School Improvement Committee

____ tutor students

FIGURE 4.12. Example of a checklist item to measure parents' involvement in their children's school.

be missed. Both authors provide sage advice. So, in specifying the time period for behavioral items, you should avoid asking respondents to recall daily or routine events (e.g., visits to the grocery store, exercise class) after a long period has passed, but the time period should be long enough to capture events occurring more rarely (e.g., graduations, births).

Guidelines for Items about Demographics (Personal Background)

Researchers frequently examine the relationship between attitudes, behaviors, and knowledge and the demographics of survey respondents. Items that address demographics collect information about respondents' backgrounds (Fink, 1995). Types of demographic information frequently collected include age, gender, income, marital status, ethnicity, and education level.

A first rule about demographics is to only ask about those characteristics that are relevant to the research questions. Respondents will at times balk at providing estimates of their income or their age. Thus, in asking for personal information, you might lose some of your respondents. So, ask yourself whether information about respondents is critical to the research.

When asking about age, ask for the precise date of birth rather than current age. Respondents' recall of current age is sometimes slightly off; so, asking for their birth date avoids this issue.

Income levels should be relevant to the respondents. Incomes of patients at a free clinic will differ from those at a private practice. To find appropriate income ranges, ask those who work with the respondents the possible income levels. Also, the time period requires consideration; thus, ask about *annual* income or *monthly* pay.

In deciding about labels to use for your demographic group, use the classification preferred by the groups responding to your survey. The *Publication Manual of the American Psychological Association* (APA, 2010) provides guidance on the use of labels. In addition, the list of ethnic groups used by the Census Bureau provides guidance in specifying demographics.

Number of Items

To this point in developing items for a survey scale, we have discussed the need to consider the relevance of the items, the audience, language, item structure, and conventions. You might ask, "How many items do I need to develop?" Fabrigar and Wood (2007) wrote that "attitudes are often multifaceted, involving cognitions, emotions, and behavioral tendencies. A single item is unlikely to capture the full scope of the attitude in question; using multiple items potentially ameliorates this problem" (p. 537).

The number of items depends on what the researcher needs to know and on how many items are needed for accurate measurement (Fink, 1995). In terms of what the researcher needs to know, the survey on transition contained six subscales: Student–Teacher Interactions, Teaching Styles, Grading Practices, Participating in Class, Getting Along with Others, and School Climate. Each subscale had between 6 and 14 items. As we shall learn in Chapter 8, to attain stable scores on a scale, the more items you have, the better. However, the number of items must be balanced with the amount of time the respondents will dedicate to the survey.

In this chapter, we focused on writing survey scale items to which study participants will respond. In Chapter 5, we discuss the choices to be made in selection of the item response scales.

FURTHER READING

Fink, A. (2003). *How to ask survey questions* (2nd ed.). Thousand Oaks, CA: Sage.

> Provides guidelines for writing survey items. Includes examples to illustrate the application of guidelines.

Peterson, R. (2000). *Constructing effective questionnaires*. Thousand Oaks, CA: Sage.

> Presents an in-depth discussion of item-writing guidelines.

CHAPTER EXERCISES

1. What revisions are needed for the item below?

My teacher uses many types of instruction activities (lecture, small-group work, computers).

2. In the item below, how should the phrase "special-needs students" be revised?

I need additional materials to teach special-needs students.

3. What is the reading level of the item below? Is the reading level appropriate for the audience?

My supervisor is responsive in addressing problems that affect my job.

4. Review the item-writing guidelines and develop an example that shows (a) the violation of a guideline in the item and (b) the same item following the guideline. Use the NOT THIS/BUT THIS form to create your example.

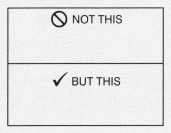

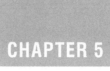

CHAPTER 5

Development of Response Scales

> *Investigators. . . . do not appear to recognise that*
> *the data they obtain will be partly dependent*
> *upon the scales and formats that they have used.*
> —HARTLEY AND BETTS (2010, p. 25)

Introduction

Just as we learned in Chapter 4 that word choices will influence survey respondents, Hartley and Betts (2010) alert us to the issue of respondents being influenced in their answers by the types of response scales that researchers use. However, researchers want any shifts in respondents' answers to be due to an intervention being implemented or the characteristics of respondents who are the focus of the study. We do not want the survey answers to change simply because of a researcher's decision to modify the order of an item response scale from "Disagree"/"Agree" to "Agree"/"Disagree." However, as we will see later in this chapter, changes in the order of the labels for **item response scales** are associated with a change in survey results. Thus, in this chapter, we focus on issues related to the development of response scales that accompany each survey item. We discuss developing item response scales that allow survey respondents to indicate (1) the direction and intensity of their attitudes, (2) the frequency of their behaviors, and (3) the depth of their understanding.

Specifically, in this chapter, we consider the length of item response scales (e.g., 1–4 or 1–6) and the use of response labels (e.g., "Strongly disagree," "Disagree," "Agree," "Strongly agree"). Also we discuss the questionable use of a middle position (e.g., "Average," "No opinion," and "Don't know") in the item response scales.

Length of the Item Response Scale

A common question asked during the development of a survey scale is "Should I use a 4-point response scale or a 5-point scale for my items?" The issue of response-scale length is critical in survey development because "with too few categories, the rating scales may fail to discriminate between respondents with different underlying judgments, whereas too many categories may make it impossible for respondents to distinguish reliably between adjacent categories" (Krebs & Hoffmeyer-Zlotnik, 2010, p. 119).

Scale Length and Purpose

In part, the answer of item length (i.e., number of response scale points) depends on whether the purpose of the items in a scale is to measure the presence or absence of a construct, respondents' depth of knowledge, or intensity of survey participants' attitudes (see Table 5.1).

Number of Response Categories and Checklists

Researchers use checklists to measure the presence or absence of a construct (e.g., skills, strategies, or behaviors). Checklists only require a blank for each item in the list. The checklist in Figure 5.1 was used to collect feedback from the staff of a family literacy program about which of the artifacts (i.e., items) in portfolios they found useful to gauge program participants' development of parenting skills. The intent of the data collection was to improve the portfolio assessment system. Based on feedback from the program staff, in subsequent years the collection and inclusion of artifacts that were informative about levels of family literacy were emphasized and less informative artifacts were deemphasized or eliminated.

TABLE 5.1. Guidelines for Addressing Scale Length

- Consider the purpose of the scale in determining response scale length.
  - Use one response category for a checklist entry.
  - Use two response categories for a knowledge item.
  - Use four or six response categories for an attitude item.
- Think about the statistical analyses to be conducted.
- Allow for the discrimination capability of respondents.
- Consider respondent preferences.

---

6. Which of the following artifacts did you find <u>most useful</u> in determining levels of family literacy? (Select and check no more than five responses.)

_____ Activities outside of Even Start: church bulletins, newsletter articles

_____ Artwork and crafts

_____ Audiotapes of parent reading to child

_____ Family Literacy Checklist

_____ Goal/planning sheets

_____ Listening Log

_____ Narratives of activities

_____ Participant calendars

_____ Participation statistics: Home Visit, Adult Basic Education/English as a Second Language, Family Literacy

_____ Photographs

_____ Portfolio Log

_____ Praise/Encouragement Log

_____ Reading Log

_____ Videotapes

_____ Writing samples

FIGURE 5.1. An example of a scale with a checklist format.

Number of Response Categories and Knowledge Items

Knowledge items require only two response categories when the respondent indicates whether a statement is true or false, myth or fact, or ethical or unethical. For example, a true–false format could be used in an instrument to measure respondents' levels of knowledge related to suicide, using items such as "Suicide is among the top 10 causes of death in the U.S." (true) and "People who talk about suicide rarely commit suicide" (false) (Hubbard & McIntosh, 1992; Segal, 2000). To examine respondents' understanding of the ways that HIV can be transmitted, Oppenheim (1992) devised a survey instrument that presented the question "How do you think AIDS is transmitted?" (p. 246). Following the question was a list of *possible* ways to transmit the virus, such as by touching someone who has the virus (not a method of transmission) and sharing needles with someone with the virus (a method of transmission). Beside each item were boxes in which the respondent selected "Yes" or "No."

Figure 5.2 shows two modified true–false items that provide two choices for respondents to select. Each item presents a brief scenario that describes classroom assessment practices that are ethical or unethical (Johnson et al., 2008). Study participants (preservice teachers, teachers, and administrators) marked the ethicality of each assessment practice. These scores provided information about the survey participants' understanding of ethical assessment practices.

5. A second-grade teacher uses observations as the sole method
students have learned.

  O Ethical

  O Unethical

6. When a child is caught cheating on a test, rather than assigning a z_.ᵤ, the
teacher gives the student an alternate version of the same test.

  O Ethical

  O Unethical

FIGURE 5.2. Items using a modified true–false format to assess educators' understanding of ethical classroom assessment practices.

Some surveys use "Do not know" or "No opinion" options for knowledge-based items (Fink, 2003). We do not recommend this response choice because research in the field of testing and measurement indicates that females are less likely than males to guess when they are uncertain about an answer (Ben-Shakhar & Sinai, 1991). We are not advocating that respondents should randomly guess; rather, if survey respondents have partial knowledge, then their understanding might best be gauged by their informed selection of an answer. If females select the "Do not know" or "No opinion" options more than their equally informed male counterparts, then scores to some extent will reflect gender **traits** rather than the construct of interest. Also, less informed examinees tend to ignore "Do not guess" instructions more often than more informed examinees; so the scores might reflect the examinee's tendency to guess rather than their actual knowledge (Wood, 1976).

Number of Response Categories and Attitude Scales

Survey items that gauge a respondent's attitude require the response scale to be more of a continuum; so the range of a scale might range from "Very unfavorable," to "Somewhat unfavorable," to "Somewhat favorable," and to "Very favorable" (see Figure 5.3). For attitude scales, researchers have suggested the use of scale points of 3–5 (Frary, 2003), 4–5 (Fink, 2003), 5–7 (Fink, 2003; Krosnick & Fabrigar, 1997), and 7–12 (Peterson, 2000).

The selection of response scale length can be informed by considering the relationship between the number of points in response scales and the consistency of scores (i.e., reliability) of an instrument. Gains in reliability level off after 5–7 scale points (Bandalos & Enders, 1996; Enders

Please tell me if you have a very favorable, somewhat favorable, somewhat unfavorable, or very unfavorable opinion of the following agencies.

Agency	Very unfavorable	Somewhat unfavorable	Somewhat favorable	Very favorable
1. Bureau of Alcohol, Tobacco and Firearms	1	2	3	4
2. Central Intelligence Agency	1	2	3	4
3. Federal Bureau of Investigation	1	2	3	4

FIGURE 5.3. Items measuring attitude toward law enforcement agencies.

& Bandalos, 1999). Similarly, in terms of the reliability of a survey scale, Lozano, García-Cueto, and Muñiz (2008) indicated four as the minimum number of response scales and seven as the maximum number of response scales.

In considering the validity associated with an instrument, Green and Rao (1970) examined the relation between the number of points on item response scales and the number of survey items in recovering a data configuration when using multidimensional scaling. They tested item-level response scales with 2, 3, 6, and 18 points and survey scales containing 4, 8, 16, and 32 items. The researchers found little improvement in recovery of the data configuration with at least 6-point item response scales and with more than eight items. Item response scales with 2 and 3 points were associated with poor recovery of the data configuration.

Statistical Analyses to Be Used with Data

Another contributing factor in making a decision about the number of response categories is the statistical analyses that will be conducted. For example, if you are interested in the differences in item means by gender, then for statistical analyses one might consider using a t-test or analysis of variance (ANOVA). However, assumptions related to normality and homogeneity of data must be tenable in using either analysis. Research studies of the robustness of t-tests and the F-test in ANOVA provide some guidance. When the dependent variable is discretely measured (e.g., 4- or 6-point scale), it appears the differences in means can be used to accurately analyze discrete data with as few as 3 points for t-tests and as few as 3–5 points for F-tests (Bevan, Denton, & Myers, 1974; Heeren & Agostino, 1987; Hsu & Feldt, 1969).

Nonparametric statistics offer an alternative to the *F*-test and the *t*-test. In a discussion of Likert scales, Barnette (2010) recommended using nonparametric analyses at the item level. Such a recommendation is supported by Nanna and Sawilowsky (1998) who compared the power of the parametric *t*-test and the nonparametric Wilcoxon rank-sum test. For a 7-point Likert-style item, the Wilcoxon test outperformed the *t*-test. In the Appendix, we provide additional discussion about deciding between parametric and nonparametric analyses.

Respondents' Discrimination Capability

In deciding on the length of item response scales, you also should take into account the discrimination capacity of the respondents. Too many scale points might result in respondents experiencing problems discriminating between the scale points and thus contributing to measurement errors (Lozano et al., 2008; Weng, 2004).

According to Frary (2003), research indicates that respondents cannot distinguish between more than six or seven response levels. Illustrating Frary's point is the response scale used by Kouzes and Posner (2002) in the Leadership Practices Inventory. Shown in Figure 5.4 is a response scale with 10 levels. However, would respondents be able to distinguish between "Seldom" and "Once in a while" or "Very frequently" and "Almost always"?

Another consideration is the age of respondents and their ability to distinguish between response levels. Will respondents be children or adults? If respondents are children, will a 2-point scale (e.g., "Disagree"/"Agree," "No"/"Yes") suffice? For example, in a survey conducted in an elementary magnet program, the students responded to items about classroom activities. One item stated, "Group work helps me to better understand my class work." Initially, the survey developers created a response scale for elementary students with the frequency categories of "Strongly disagree," "Disagree," "Agree," and "Strongly agree." The faculty at the elementary school, however, requested a "Yes"/"No" response scale for their students to avoid confusion. Responding to a 4-point scale appeared daunting for elementary students. Responding required students to read a statement, determine the direction of their response ("Disagree"/"Agree"), and decide the extent (i.e., "Disagree" or "Strongly disagree"; "Agree" or "Strongly agree") to which they agreed with the statement.

---

1) Almost never; 2) Rarely; 3) Seldom; 4) Once in a while; 5) Occasionally;
6) Sometimes; 7) Fairly often; 8) Usually; 9) Very frequently; 10) Almost always

---

FIGURE 5.4. A response scale that requires a high capacity of respondent discrimination.

Respondent Preferences

A final consideration is that of respondent preference. In a study of the use of a two-choice response scale versus a six-choice response scale, respondents expressed greater acceptance of the six-choice version (Velicer, DiClemente, & Corriveau, 1984).

There is, however, too much of a good thing. Indicating that little was to be gained with lengthy scales, Dawes (2008) found that the average number of scale points that respondents used for a 5-point response scale was 2.9 (58%); for a 7-point scale, 3.6 (51%); and for a 10-point scale, 4.0 (40%). In this instance, as response scale points increased, respondents used a lower percentage of the points.

Numeric and Verbal Response Labels

Should you use a numeric scale with your survey items? Should your item response scale use verbal labels (e.g., "Never," "Sometimes," "Always," "All the time")? Should you order your response scale from negative to positive (e.g., "Disagree" to "Agree") or positive to negative ("Agree" to "Disagree")? This section examines the issues in the use of numeric and verbal labels in response scales.

Numeric and Verbal Labels

The response scales for each item should use numeric and verbal labels (see Table 5.2). In marketing, for example, it is common to use both numerical and verbal labels on all points of an item response scale (Peterson, 1997). Tradition is not the only reason for using both verbal and numeric labels.

TABLE 5.2. Guidelines for Numeric and Verbal Response Labels

- Use numeric and verbal labels.
- Label all response categories.
- Develop labels to be consistent with the purpose of the scale.
- Write labels for the two endpoints that mean the opposite of each other.
- Use positive integers for numeric labels.
- Consider the effect of bias and the extremes of the scale.
- Write labels to reflect equal intervals along a continuum.
- Order the response scales from negative to positive.
- Arrange the response options in a logical order.

Adding verbal anchors has been associated with an increase in reliability (Bendig, 1953, 1954). Not all developers of surveys agree with the use of numeric and verbal labels. Based on a review of the literature on developing survey scales, Krosnick and Fabrigar (1997) recommended using verbal labels for all scale points but avoiding numeric values altogether.

Labels for Response Categories

In writing an item response scale, you should label all of the response categories (Krosnick & Fabrigar, 1997; Maitland, 2009). Maitland (2009) advised that "the approach to labeling should be the one that most clearly defines the response scale for respondents" (para. 2). When labels are used for response scales with 7–8 scale points, score consistency is higher (Weng, 2004).

An advantage of specifying anchor labels for every scale point is facilitating the interpretation of survey results (Weng, 2004). Figure 5.5 illustrates the issue. If you are reporting the quality of services at a health clinic and the mean is 3.4, interpretation of the finding is difficult when using the top scale with only the endpoints labeled. Do you indicate that respondents considered the quality of services as "Good" or "Very good"? When you have every scale point labeled, as is the case in the bottom scale, the interpretation is more straightforward. In this instance, the 3.4 means respondents consider the quality of services to be "Good," not "Very good."

Labels and the Purpose of the Scale

Types of response options include frequency, endorsement, quality, intensity, and comparison (Fink, 2003; Peterson, 2000). Examples of verbal labels used in response scales include those shown in Table 5.3. Notice

⃠ NOT THIS			
Quality of Services	Very		Very
Doctor's sensitivity to cultural	poor		good
background	1	2 3	4
✓ BUT THIS			
Quality of Services	Very		Very
Doctor's sensitivity to cultural	poor	Poor Good	good
background	1	2 3	4

FIGURE 5.5. Labeling all response categories.

TABLE 5.3. Examples of Numeric and Verbal Labels in Item Response Scales

Types	Scales				
	4-point response scales				
Frequency	Never 1	Seldom 2	Often 3	All the time 4	
Endorsement	Very unfavorable 1	Unfavorable 2	Favorable 3	Very favorable 4	
Endorsement	Strongly disapprove 1	Disapprove 2	Approve 3	Strongly approve 4	
Endorsement	Not important at all 1	Unimportant 2	Important 3	Very important 4	
Quality	Poor 1	Fair 2	Good 3	Excellent 4	
	6-point response scales				
Intensity	Strongly disagree 1	Disagree 2	Slightly disagree 3	Slightly agree 4	Agree 5	Strongly agree 6
Frequency	Never 1	Rarely 2	Occasionally 3	Fairly often 4	Very often 5	All the time 6
Endorsement	Strongly oppose 1	Oppose 2	Somewhat oppose 3	Somewhat favor 4	Favor 5	Strongly favor 6
Endorsement	Very unlikely 1	Somewhat unlikely 2	Slightly unlikely 3	Slightly likely 4	Somewhat likely 5	Very likely 6
Quality	Very poor 1	Poor 2	Fair 3	Good 4	Very good 5	Excellent 6
Quality	Worst possible problem 1	Very serious problem 2	Severe problem 3	Moderate problem 4	Minor problem 5	No problem 6

that different labels serve different purposes. Labels such as "Never"/"All the time" can be used to gauge the frequency of respondents' behaviors; whereas labels of "Very unfavorable"/"Very favorable" are appropriate to use with an attitude scale in which respondents are endorsing positions of a political party or statements related to a bond issue.

Do not make the mistake of using a scale that does not gauge the construct being measured. As shown in Figure 5.6, in some instances, researchers will use "Disagree"/"Agree" labels with survey items that gauge behavior. However, if you are gauging parental involvement in the classroom, then the response scale should be related to frequency. In such an instance, the response scale should use labels related to the frequency of a behavior, such as Daily, Weekly, Monthly, and Once or twice a year. Incorrect use of labels can result in data that are not interpretable. For example, if parents disagree with the top item in Figure 5.6 about occasionally volunteering in their child's classroom, do we interpret their response to mean they rarely volunteer or they frequently volunteer?

Labels for Two Endpoints That Mean the Opposite of Each Other

A starting point in writing an item response scale is to develop two endpoints that mean the opposite of each other (Fink, 2003). As shown in Table 5.3, for the concept of frequency the endpoints might be "Never" and "All the time." For the concept of endorsement, the endpoints might be "Strongly oppose" and "Strongly favor." With the endpoints selected, you can use the examples in Table 5.3 to fill in the middle labels.

		🚫 NOT THIS				
I occasionally volunteer in my child's classroom.	Strongly disagree 1	Disagree 2	Slightly disagree 3	Slightly agree 4	Agree 5	Strongly agree 6
		✓ BUT THIS				
How often do you volunteer in your child's classroom?	Not able to volunteer 1	Once or twice a year 2	Monthly 3	Weekly 4	Daily 5	

FIGURE 5.6. An example of the need for the labels in item response scales to be consistent with the construct.

Positive Integers for Numeric Labels

The numeric values used in item response scales influence survey participants' selection of response options (Mazaheri & Theuns, 2009; Schwarz,
Knäuper, Hippler, Noelle-Neumann, & Clark, 1991; Tourangeau, Couper,
& Conrad, 2007). When items were labeled on the endpoints only (e.g., "Not
at all satisfied"/"Very satisfied" and "Not at all successful"/"Extremely
successful"), the choice of numeric labels influenced respondents' choices.
Consider the case of item response scales with endpoint labels accompanied
with numeric response scales of −5 to +5 and 1 to 10. The percentage of
respondents in the bottom half of the scale differed for the two types of
scales (Mazaheri & Theuns, 2009; Schwarz et al., 1991). For the −5 to 5
scale, fewer responses occurred in the bottom half (−5 to 0) than occurred
in the bottom (1 to 5) of the 1–10 scale. That is, the use of negative numeric
values shifted responses toward the high end of the scale. This finding is a
reminder of the importance of clarity in the language of a survey. Schwarz
et al. (1991) noted that " 'Not at all successful' may be interpreted as referring to the absence of success if combined with a numeric value of 0, but
as referring to the presence of explicit failure if combined with a numeric
value of −5" (p. 572). Tourangeau et al. (2007) reported similar results
when using a 7-point scale that ranged from −3 to +3.

The Effect of Bias and Scale Extremes

The specific response alternatives offered can significantly influence
respondents' answers (Wright, Gaskell, & O'Muircheartaigh, 1994). In the
study of Wright et al., respondents were asked how many hours they spent
watching television and the response options discriminated at low or high
frequency. Labels for the low-frequency condition were as follows:

> Less than half an hour
> Half an hour but less than 1 hour
> 1 hour but less than 1½ hours
> 1½ hours but less than 2 hours
> 2 hours but less than 2½ hours
> 2½ hours or more

For the high-frequency condition, the response alternatives were
labeled as follows:

> Less than 2½ hours
> 2½ hours but less than 3 hours
> 3 hours but less than 3½ hours

3½ hours but less than 4 hours

4 hours but less than 4½ hours

4½ hours or more

When the response options discriminated more finely at low viewing levels, approximately 20% fewer respondents indicated they watch 2½ hours or more a day. That is, when presented with an option that presented 2½ hours of television viewing as an extreme value, respondents might have underreported their actual television viewing. One possible remedy is conducting a focus group to investigate the response options that offer respondents an appropriate range of options.

Labels to Reflect Equal Intervals along a Continuum

The labels in the response scales should reflect equal intervals along a continuum (Fink, 2003; Krosnick & Fabrigar, 1997), and the answer choices along the continuum should be balanced to avoid building in bias (Peterson, 2000). An example of bias is shown in Figure 5.7. Note that the top response scale has two levels that indicate the reasons for selection of a graduate school are not important (i.e., "Not at all important" and

	NOT THIS				
Reasons for Selecting a Community College	Two levels			Three levels	
	Not at all important	**Somewhat important**	**Important**	**Very important**	**Extremely important**
Career paths	1	2	3	4	5
Financial aid	1	2	3	4	5
Proximity to work	1	2	3	4	5
	BUT THIS				
Reasons for Selecting a Community College	Two levels		Two levels		
	Not at all important	**Somewhat unimportant**	**Somewhat important**	**Very important**	
Career paths	1	2	3	4	
Financial aid	1	2	3	4	
Proximity to work	1	2	3	4	

FIGURE 5.7. An example of unbalanced and balanced response scales.

"Somewhat important"). In contrast, the scale has three levels indicating that the reason for selection is important (i.e., "Important," "Very important," and "Extremely important"). Thus, the mean for each item is likely to be positively biased. The bottom scale has balance with two levels of not important and two levels of important.

Order of Response Scales: Negative to Positive

Barnette (2010) and Fink (2003) advised that the order of scale points move from negative to positive. Research supports the ordering of response scales from negative to positive. As with the example shown in Figure 5.8, when a positive label or a high rating is used on the left of a response scale, the means for the survey items are higher than the means for items that begin with a negative label ("Strongly disagree") or rating (Hartley & Betts, 2010; Krebs & Hoffmeyer-Zlotnik, 2010; Nicholls, Orr, Okubo, & Loftus, 2006). Nicholls and colleagues reported that "Definitely agree" statements were inflated by 27% when favorable response scale points were on the left side. Such a bias holds true for adults and for children when either a positive label or a high numeric value is presented on the left (Betts & Hartley, 2012). Beginning items with negative labels, however, was not associated with a lower mean (Krebs & Hoffmeyer-Zlotnik, 2010).

A consequence of a positive bias is evident when survey scales are used to make absolute decisions. This occurs, for example, when an agency sets an annual performance goal to achieve an overall mean of 3 on a 4-point client satisfaction scale. Then, the placement of the favorable response scale

		⊘ NOT THIS			
Very satisfied	Satisfied	Somewhat satisfied	Somewhat dissatisfied	Dissatisfied	Very dissatisfied
6	5	4	3	2	1

		⊘ NOR THIS			
Very satisfied	Very dissatisfied	Satisfied	Dissatisfied	Somewhat satisfied	Somewhat dissatisfied
1	2	3	4	5	6

		✓ BUT THIS			
Very dissatisfied	Dissatisfied	Somewhat dissatisfied	Somewhat satisfied	Satisfied	Very satisfied
1	2	3	4	5	6

FIGURE 5.8. Order for response scales.

points on the left will inflate the overall mean and overestimate client satisfaction.

Response Options in a Logical Order

Placement of response options in a logical order influences survey participants' response time (Tourangeau, Couper, & Conrad, 2004). In their investigation, Tourangeau and colleagues arranged response options vertically, with one version arranged arbitrarily from bottom to top as "Disagree," "Agree," "Strongly disagree," "Strongly agree," and "It depends." Another response scale was arranged in the expected order of "Strongly disagree," "Disagree," "It depends," "Agree," and "Strongly agree." When faced with labels in an unexpected order, respondents answered more slowly than when responding to the response scale with labels in the expected order. Although this might appear to be a minor issue, a researcher wants to keep a respondent's cognitive load minimal to reduce fatigue and avoid the respondent terminating the survey.

The Questionable Middle Position

Much debate surrounds the use of a middle position in a Likert-type response scale. In addition, it is not always clear what constitutes a middle position. Do middle positions include the response categories of "Neutral," "Don't know," "No opinion," and "Average"? In this section, we review the research on the use of middle positions in survey scales.

Even Number of Response Categories to Avoid Neutral Responses

Fink's (2003) position on the use of odd or even scales was that no conclusive evidence supports the use of either scale. As stated in Table 5.4, an advantage of response scales with an even number of options is that they avoid a neutral response (Peterson, 2000). Fink (2003) described a neutral category as a middle point (e.g., neither happy nor unhappy) or a "No opinion"/"Don't know" option. We often use rating scales to discriminate between respondents with different underlying judgments (Krebs & Hoffmeyer-Zlotnik, 2010, p. 119). For example, we write survey items to measure parents' participation in school events (i.e., behavior) and health care providers' job satisfaction (i.e., attitudes). If potential survey respondents are likely to vary in these dimensions—for example, some health care providers being satisfied with their job responsibilities, whereas others are not—then survey items need to discriminate (i.e., distinguish) between those satisfied with their job and those who are not. Allowing a middle

TABLE 5.4. Guidelines for Neutral Positions

- Use an even number of response categories to avoid neutral responses.

- Consider a response scale with an odd number of categories when gauging the quality of a service or the status quo.

- Offer moderating options (e.g., "somewhat," "slightly") when using a middle option.

- Avoid use of the "Don't know" option; however, consider its use if uninformed respondents might provide faulty information because they feel pressured to answer.

- Provide "Don't know" when using unfamiliar options.

- Set nonsubstantive options (e.g., "Don't know," "No opinion," "Does not apply," or "Cannot respond") apart from the other response options.

position might "muddy the waters" and prevent researchers from discriminating between those, for example, satisfied with services and respondents not satisfied with services.

Odd Number of Response Categories for Quality or to Support the Status Quo

With all this said, at times a middle position is required. In Figure 5.9, the item required a middle response that allows respondents to compare two forms of instruction: face to face and online. In comparing the quality of two or more modes of instruction, respondents might legitimately indicate the outcomes, for the forms of learning are the same.

The item in Figure 5.10 required a middle response that expresses support for the status quo, that is, maintain the same amount of homework. The issue is not whether or not respondents support homework, but rather respondents' perceptions about the amount of homework.

As can be seen in these two examples, the middle position is not always a "Neutral" or "No opinion." Other examples of middle positions assess

Compared to face-to-face learning, outcomes from online learning are currently . . .	1 Inferior	2 Somewhat inferior	3 The same	4 Somewhat superior	5 Superior

FIGURE 5.9. Item that requires the middle position to measure quality. Adapted from Allen and Seaman (2006).

The amount of homework for this course was . . .	1 Too little	2 Reasonable	3 Too great

FIGURE 5.10. An item that requires the middle position to gauge status quo. Adapted from Frary (2003).

respondents' perceptions about (1) whether penalties for breaking the law should be "More strict," "About the same as now," or "Less strict"; (2) the amount of foreign aid is "Too much," "The right amount," or "Not enough"; (3) the control of the federal government over local education is "Too much," "The right amount," or "Too little"; and (4) obtaining a divorce should be "Easier," "Stay as is," or "Be more difficult" (Schuman & Presser, 1996).

Moderating Options When Using a Middle Option

Presser and Schuman (1980) reported that when a middle position was explicitly offered in interviews, the percentage of respondents choosing such an option was higher than for respondents for whom a middle position was not explicitly offered. Offering survey participants response options that reflected moderate views (i.e., "Somewhat liberal" and "Somewhat conservative") shifted respondents away from the middle position. For example, when presented with the options of "Liberal," "Conservative," or "Middle of the road" a higher percentage of respondents selected "Middle of the road." In contrast, respondents less often selected the "Middle of the road" option when offered moderating alternatives, such as "Liberal," "Somewhat liberal," "Middle of the road," "Somewhat conservative," or "Conservative."

"Don't Know" and "No Opinion"

An important consideration in using a "Don't know" (DK) option is that its absence possibly encourages respondents to provide faulty information. Bishop, Tuchfarber, and Oldendick (1986) reported that in interview surveys the respondents were much more likely to offer an opinion on a fictitious issue when the question was asked without a DK option than when a DK filter was asked with the question. The authors conjectured that respondents give opinions on fictitious issues due to pressure to answer.

Higher reliability (i.e., score consistency) is an advantage of "Agree"/"Disagree" response scales with 4 points and 6 points and no middle position as compared to response scales with 5 and 7 points that used an "Undecided" option as a midpoint (Masters, 1974). Based on their review of the literature, Krosnick and Fabrigar (1997) recommended against offering the "No opinion" (NO) option. They tempered their recommendation by noting that the use might be required when the issues are obscure.

Francis and Busch (1975) tested the hypothesis that DK and NO responses are a nonrandom phenomenon. That is, they examined whether these responses were systematically related to respondent characteristics. They found that females were more likely than males to give DK or NO responses. Selection of these responses also differed by race, education, and income. Thus, to avoid bias, researchers should be careful to include these respondents in their analyses and examine the responses for the subgroups (Francis & Busch, 1975).

DK and Unfamiliar Options

Another issue related to respondents' knowledge is their answers being influenced by the position of unfamiliar options within a survey item. Respondents' answers about an unfamiliar item, such as the type of car, were influenced by the position of the items in a list of cars (Tourangeau et al., 2004). The authors reported that when respondents were asked to indicate whether or not several makes and models of cars were expensive, the answers for the unfamiliar items depended on the other types of cars that were nearby on the list. In such a case, the DK option might be needed to avoid respondent tendency to answer an item to meet the researcher's expectations.

Nonsubstantive Options Set Apart from the Other Response Options

On the occasion when a DK or NO is required, you need to determine where to place the option in relation to the item response scale. That is, do you put the DK or NO option in the middle of the scale? Do you put the option at the end of the response scale? Or, do you place the option adjacent to the item response scale but not as part of the scale? Does it make a difference? The placement of "No opinion" and "Don't know" options in the response scale has influenced responses (Tourangeau et al., 2004). In a response scale, when substantive options (e.g., "Disagree," "Agree"; "Unfavorable," "Favorable") were not differentiated from the nonsubstantive options of DK and NO, the respondents tended to use the visual rather than the conceptual midpoint. Thus, in Figure 5.11, "Agree slightly" becomes the midpoint and is associated with a shift of responses to the higher end of the scale. The authors recommended the DK and NO options should be separated from the response options. Similarly, Barnette (2010) recommended that the nonsubstantive options "Does not apply" and "Cannot respond" should not be placed within the response continuum.

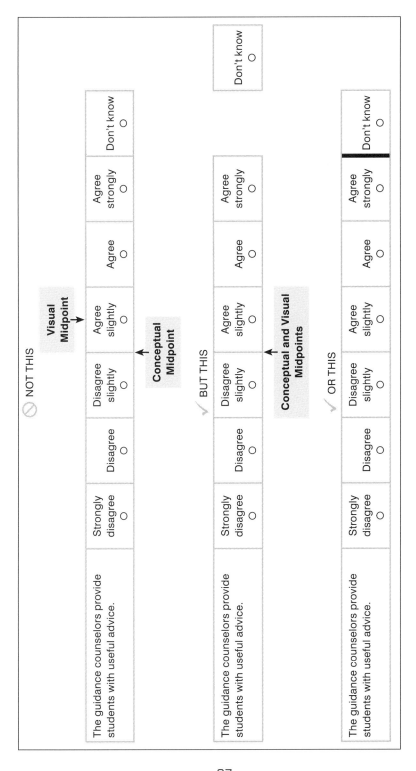

FIGURE 5.11. Formatting nonsubstantive options apart from the other response options.

87

Tourangeau et al. (2004) examined the effect of the placement of the "It depends" option. As shown below, the options were formatted vertically, and the "It depends" option was placed in the middle of the response scale and at the end of the scale.

Strongly agree	Strongly agree
Agree	Agree
It depends	Disagree
Disagree	Strongly disagree
Strongly disagree	It depends

Respondents were more likely to select the neutral "It depends" option when it came in the middle of the scale. Thus, placement of "It depends" and other neutral responses should be at the bottom of vertically formatted response scales.

We close this chapter with a quote from Schwarz et al. (1991): "Far from being 'neutral measurement devices,' the response alternatives that are provided to respondents do constitute a source of information that respondents actively use in determining their task and in constructing a reasonable answer" (p. 578). In Chapter 6, we discuss the selection of the survey format (e.g., website or pencil and paper), offer some guidelines specific to formatting items in a **protocol,** and establish the need to complete reviews of the survey scale.

FURTHER READING

Fink, A. (2003). *How to ask survey questions* (2nd ed.). Thousand Oaks, CA: Sage.

> *Discusses the development of response scales. Includes examples to illustrate the application of guidelines.*

Peterson, R. (2000). *Constructing effective questionnaires*. Thousand Oaks, CA: Sage.

> *Presents an in-depth discussion of developing response scales.*

CHAPTER EXERCISES

1. You want to know the activities in which socially engaged students participate. A partial list is shown below. Which type of response scale should be used: checklist, true–false, or Likert style?

   Academic clubs (such as business, debate, DECA, Latin, Spanish, French, and science competitions)

   Athletic programs (such as baseball, basketball, cheerleading, cross country/track, football, golf, soccer, softball, tennis, volleyball, and wrestling)

   Service clubs (such as ADAPT, Anchor Club, Civitan, Key Club, and SADD)

2. What type of response scale is used in the following item?

Would you recommend your health plan to your friends?	Definitely not ○	Probably not ○	Probably yes ○	Definitely yes ○

3. For items 3a to 3c, indicate what change should be made to the response scale of each item.

a.

I visit the fitness gym weekly.	Strongly disagree 1	Disagree 2	Agree 3	Strongly agree 4

b.

Ease of making appointment through our website.	Poor 1	Fair 2	Good 3	Very good 4	Excellent 5

c.

Students receive a more advanced learning experience at the Center for Knowledge than they would at their regularly assigned schools.	Disagree strongly ○	Disagree ○	Do not know ○	Agree ○	Agree strongly ○

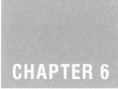

CHAPTER 6

Formatting and Reviewing

Measure twice, cut once.
—CARPENTERS' PROVERB

Introduction

The translation of this long-standing advice from carpenters is to "plan and prepare in a careful, thorough manner before taking action" (Wikipedia, 2016). To this point, you have expended resources to develop items and item-level response scales that appear to address your research focus. However, before you rush to administer these items, your planning and preparation should include selecting the most appropriate format for the survey (e.g., pencil and paper or web page) and, critically, submitting the draft instrument to a review process. This review process should include a pilot of the instrument with a group of respondents similar to those who will complete the operational survey. In this chapter, we consider the selection of the survey format and offer some guidelines specific to formatting items in the survey instrument. We conclude the chapter with a discussion about the need to complete reviews of the survey instrument.

Survey Format and Administration Method

In formatting the survey, one option to consider is whether data are best collected through the use of a self-administered instrument or an interview. Formats of self-administered surveys include pencil-and-paper questionnaires completed individually or in group settings, mail surveys, and web pages (see Figure 6.1). Other options include face-to-face and telephone interviews as well as focus groups. In the column header of Figure 6.1, we

Formats	Types	Low cost	Short timeframe	Large number of respondents	Low writing demands	Attractive protocol	Probing	Clarification of respondents' questions	Explore alternative views	Confidentiality/ anonymity	Low data entry demands
SELF-ADMINISTERED INSTRUMENTS	Questionnaire: self-administration	✓	✓	✓		✓				✓	
	Questionnaire: self-administration in a group setting	✓	✓	✓		✓		✓		✓	
	Mail			✓		✓				✓	
	Web	✓	✓	✓		✓				✓	✓
INTERVIEWS	Face to face				✓		✓	✓	✓	✓	
	Focus group		✓		✓		✓	✓	✓		
	Telephone interview				✓		✓	✓	✓	✓	

FIGURE 6.1. Advantages of survey formats. Based on Fink (2013), Fowler (2014), Goddard and Villanova (2006), Nathan (2008), Solomon (2001), and Sue and Ritter (2012).

list the qualities that should inform your selection of the methods for survey administration.

Cost

In terms of cost, the self-administered formats will be relatively less expensive as compared to interview methods. This is in part due to the need for an interviewer or the need for a moderator in the case of focus groups.

Timeframe

As shown in Figure 6.1, a short timeframe for a study is possible for questionnaires, web surveys, and focus groups. Mail surveys require a longer timeframe to allow for the delivery of the surveys and their return posting. Face-to-face and telephone interviews require making arrangements for a time to conduct each interview and the time commitment for completing each interview. This contrasts with a one-time meeting for a focus group.

Number of Respondents

The self-administered survey formats, such as pencil-and-paper questionnaires and web surveys, can be used with a large number of survey participants. In contrast, fewer respondents can be surveyed when data collection involves interviews or focus groups.

Writing Demands

Writing demands are reduced for respondents participating in an interview format. The interviewer can ask the survey questions and adjust when the respondent does not appear to understand the questions. In contrast, any open-response items in self-administered forms might make unwelcome demands on respondents' writing capabilities.

Attractive Protocol

Pencil-and-paper questionnaires and web page instruments can be attractively formatted with the use of graphics and color. The web-based survey also offers the possibility of video and audio features.

Follow-Up on a Response

A common strength of interview formats is that they allow a researcher to follow up on a response. The researcher can probe unexpected responses, clarify respondents' statements, answer respondents' questions, and explore alternative lines of questioning. In contrast, the items in printed and web surveys typically are standardized, predetermined questions and follow-up questions that are asked of all respondents.

Anonymity/Confidentiality

Anonymity is possible for self-administered formats only. Anonymity requires that a respondent's identity not be connected with his or her responses. Even if the researcher is the only member of the survey team who can link the identity of survey participants with the responses each provided, the survey participants' answers are not anonymous. However, if the survey responses are not associated with the respondents' name and if data are restricted access, then maintaining confidentiality of responses is plausible. Confidentiality can be maintained across administration formats with the exception of focus groups. A challenge associated with focus groups is that members of a focus group might make public the views expressed by individual members. Thus, focus groups do not appear to offer confidentiality.

Data Entry

A great benefit of web-based surveys is that data entry is generally eliminated. Web applications typically have a function that exports survey responses to a database, such as Excel or IBM SPSS Statistics Software (SPSS)[1], for statistical analyses.

Item Formats
Specific to Administration Methods

As the development of a survey comes to an end, the items must be formatted and positioned within the survey instrument. In this section, we discuss item formats specific to administration methods (see Table 6.1).

Equal Spacing of the Response Options on Print and Web Surveys

In print and web-based surveys, equal spacing of response options will avoid the introduction of bias. When spacing of the response options is varied, as in Figure 6.2, Tourangeau et al. (2004) reported that survey responses were closer to the visual midpoint than the conceptual midpoint. In Figure 6.2, this means that if "agree" is shifted toward the visual midpoint, it is likely to be selected more often than when the scale has even spacing.

---

[1]SPSS® Inc. was acquired by IBM® in 2009. IBM, the IBM logo, *ibm.com*, and SPSS are registered trademarks of International Business Machines Corporation.

TABLE 6.1. Guidelines for Formatting

- Use equal spacing of the response options to avoid the introduction of bias.
- Place each item on its own screen if the survey will be computer-based.
- Use radio buttons for respondents to indicate their response for computer-based surveys.
- Position scales horizontally.
- Use the same color (e.g., shades of blue) across the response continuum, rather than different colors for the low end of the response scale (e.g., shades of red) and the high end of the scale (e.g., shades of blue).

Further insight into spacing is provided by Smith (1995). In a survey item about social stratification, 59.8% of the respondents in the Netherlands indicated they were in the middle position of a social ranking scale, whereas the other countries (i.e., Australia, Italy, Germany, the United States, Switzerland, Austria, Great Britain, and Hungary) ranged from 72.2 to 83.8%. Such a striking difference prompted further investigation of the results. Response scales were designed to have 10 vertically stacked, equally sized boxes with the lowest labeled "Bottom" and the highest labeled "Top." The correct format was used with all the countries except for the Dutch response scale. The Dutch scale was a pyramid, with wider boxes at the bottom. The authors indicated that respondents may have been attracted to the lower boxes because they were wider and were probably perceived as indicating the social ranking of most people.

NOT THIS

	Strongly disagree	Disagree	Disagree slightly	Agree slightly	Agree	Agree strongly
It is fair to limit students' privileges here at school when their grades are too low.	O	O	O	O	O	O

BUT THIS

	Strongly disagree	Disagree	Disagree slightly	Agree slightly	Agree	Agree strongly
It is fair to limit students' privileges here at school when their grades are too low.	O	O	O	O	O	O

FIGURE 6.2. Use of equal spacing in formatting response categories.

Each Item on Its Own Screen: Computer-Based Surveys

For web-based surveys, another consideration in formatting is whether multiple items are displayed on a screen or whether each item is presented on its own screen (Couper, Traugott, & Lamias, 2001; Tourangeau et al., 2004). Such a concern is relevant when separating items across several screens might be necessary if the number of items prevents the use of one screen.

Responses to items proved to be more consistently similar among items appearing together on a screen than items separated across several screens (Couper et al., 2001; Tourangeau et al., 2004). In addition, Tourangeau et al. (2004) reported that respondents who answered the items listed on a single screen showed less differentiation in their responses to reverse-worded items than those who received items on two screens or on eight screens.

Radio Buttons for Responding on Web-Based Surveys

With web surveys, radio buttons or entry boxes can be used to provide responses. To examine the quality of information from web surveys that use radio buttons or entry boxes, Couper et al. (2001) developed a web-based item in which respondents indicated the racial/ethnic groups of 10 friends with whom they socialized most. Groups included White/Caucasian, African American, Asian, Hispanic, and other. The researchers found that entry box versions were associated with more missing data than radio buttons. However, those actually completing the entry box were more likely to provide answers that summed to 10 across the groups.

Horizontally Positioning Response Scales on Print and Web Surveys

Should response scales be positioned vertically or horizontally? Mazaheri and Theuns (2009) found that the horizontal and vertical response scale formats provided similar means when only endpoints were labeled. However, if respondents were to make judgments about the qualities of target items, such as the cost of living in a list of cities, then when options were listed *vertically*, respondents tended to rate the cities at the top of the list higher than the cities at the bottom of the list (Tourangeau et al., 2004). Thus, to avoid bias with vertical scales, it appears preferable to position response scales horizontally.

Color and the Continuum of the Response Scale

With web-based surveys, the use of color on response scales can make the survey more attractive. However, Tourangeau et al. (2007) found that when the endpoints of the scale were shaded in different colors, the responses tended to shift toward the high end of the scale, as compared to scales in which both ends of the scale were shades of the same color. The effect of color was eliminated when each scale point had a verbal or numerical label.

Complete Reviews and a Pilot of the Survey Scale

As a final step in the development of the survey scale, the instrument should pass through several reviews. Potential reviewers of the survey include subject matter experts, survey methodologists, translators, copyeditors, and diversity representatives.

Subject Matter Expert Review

A subject matter expert can provide feedback about the match between the survey items and the construct that is the focus of the survey scale. The content expert can also provide feedback about whether any facets of the construct are not represented in the survey scale and whether some facets are overrepresented. Such a review also informs the researcher about whether the language is appropriate to the current conceptualization of the construct measured by the survey. The review will provide content validity evidence about the accuracy of the inferences we make based on the survey results.

Survey Methodologist Review

A reviewer with expertise in survey development can provide feedback about the item stems and response scales. The survey methodologist can also review the formatting of the survey instrument.

Translator Review

If the survey is to be translated into another language, then the translation should be reviewed by potential respondents who are fluent in the language. For example, surveys that have been translated for English language learners should be reviewed by members of the language community. Assuming the translated surveys reflect the intent of the English version of the survey is perhaps unwarranted. Thus, a survey will benefit from translation done by a member of the language community who did not serve on the survey development team.

Editorial Review

Editorial reviews also contribute to the quality of surveys. An editorial review will support the clarity of the items and remove any errors of language conventions that detract from the professional look of the survey protocol.

Bias Review

A review for bias will help to ensure that survey participants' answers reflect the intent of the items and not participants' reactions to offensive wording or stereotypical depiction of groups. Members of the review committee should be representative of those who will be the focus of the survey study.

Conducting a Pilot Test

Conducting a **pilot test** is part of the review process. The pilot should be conducted in a context similar to the planned administration. The pilot will provide information about whether the respondents will be able to complete the survey and if they are likely to provide accurate information.

Participants in the pilot should be similar to those who will complete the operational survey. For instance, a survey planned for administration to students would benefit from a small pilot conducted with a group of students demographically similar to those targeted for the survey. As part of the pilot, this select group of respondents both completes the survey instrument (e.g., web page or paper-and-pencil questionnaire) and provides feedback about the items. The survey developer should ask questions about pilot group members' understanding of the items and their ability to answer questions. Feedback from the pilot group about their experience in completing the survey allows you to determine if the language in the items is relevant; if any wording is offensive; if the survey items are clear; if the item scales were difficult to understand; and if important issues were omitted. The pilot also will inform you about the time required to complete the survey, determining whether it is too long and should be shortened. The completed surveys should be collected and used to examine whether the format creates any confusion, such as whether respondents are omitting or incorrectly responding to sections of the instrument.

Pilot testing the administration format is important. For example, did the respondents who field-tested a web survey experience problems with the browser? Did the mail surveys arrive in the designated timeframe for the survey timeline? Did members of the focus group identify other items that should be added to the protocol that will be used in the study?

Feedback from the reviews and the pilot test should be compiled and changes made to reflect the suggested revisions. After the changes are complete, in a next step a field test can be conducted to examine the statistical quality of the survey scale. We discuss the conduct of a field test in Chapter

8. In Chapter 7, we present statistical methods that will be useful in reviewing the quality of the items and the reliability and validity associated with the scale.

FURTHER READING

Tourangeau, R., Conrad, F., & Couper, M. (2013). *The science of web surveys.* New York: Oxford University Press.

> *Provides an in-depth treatment of the use of web surveys in the survey process.*

CHAPTER EXERCISES

1. Which survey format (e.g., web-based, interviews, paper and pencil) is most suitable for a survey that contains multiple scales with Likert-style items?

2. Provide an example of a survey in which responses are anonymous and an instance in which responses are confidential.

3. We stated that the participants in a pilot study should be similar to those who will complete the operational survey. You plan to conduct a survey with ninth-grade students about their career interests. All ninth-grade students will complete the operational survey. To pilot the test, you plan to ask a group of 10 students in eighth grade to complete the instrument and give you feedback. Will the pilot likely provide useful information about the instrument?

CHAPTER 7

Analysis of Survey Scale Data

. . . . and the time may not be very remote when it will be
understood that for complete initiation as an efficient citizen . . . ,
it is as necessary to be able to compute, to think in averages and
maxima and minima, as it is now to be able to read and write.

—WELLS (1904, p. 192)

Introduction

Just as we use surveys to gauge the condition of our community, we also use statistics to inform us about our school, agency, or business. Another important application of statistics is to investigate the quality of research instruments, such as survey scales. In Chapter 7, we present methods of conducting descriptive analyses of data from survey scales. Examples will demonstrate the use of frequencies and measures of central tendency (i.e., mean, **median**, and **mode**) and spread (i.e., **variance**, **standard deviation**, and **range**) to describe the data at the item, scale, and subscale levels. Examining the correlation between the survey scale and other research variables will be presented. The chapter will also guide readers in interpreting the results of descriptive analyses.

To begin our discussion, imagine being asked by a large school district to develop a survey about its students' perceptions of the quality of their education, their awareness of opportunities for higher education, and their understanding about the educational requirements of various career paths. In order to collect this information from the largest number of students possible, a 30-item survey will be developed for data collection. As part of the development, you plan to field-test the survey scale with a sample of the district's 30,000 high school students. One out of every six students is randomly selected for inclusion in the field test of the survey. After the

5,000 completed surveys are returned, the data are compiled into a database. How do you go about summarizing the student responses to examine the descriptive qualities of the items and scale? The statistical procedures we present in this chapter will help answer this question.

As a discipline characterized by the analysis and summary of data, statistics is often conceptualized as having two major areas: descriptive and inferential. An extensive treatment of the use of inferential statistics and survey scales is included in the Appendix. Here we focus on descriptive statistics and their use in describing characteristics of a sample.

In this chapter, we present a variety of descriptive statistics that are likely to be applied in the investigation of survey data. In addition, we outline the data considerations associated with each statistic. The reader will also be introduced to the levels of measurement and measures of central tendency, spread, and association.

Levels of Measurement

Different types of data provide varying amounts of information and can be classified based on the amount of information they contain. The classification scheme is referred to as the levels of measurement and categorizes data as nominal, ordinal, interval, and ratio. An understanding of the levels of data is critical because statistical analyses are specific to each level.

Nominal Data

In addition to the scales included in surveys, researchers often want to collect demographic information about respondents. Consider "gender," for example. A survey researcher might use the demographic variable of gender to investigate the possibility of item bias by employing a statistical procedure that examines whether females and males with a similar overall ability or trait, such as attitude toward writing, display, on average, systematically different responses to a particular item (AERA et al., 2014, p. 16). Therefore, survey participants may be asked to report such demographics as gender, ethnic background, marital status, school name, or similar descriptive classifications.

Demographic information is considered nominal or categorical data. No underlying order or structure exists in the categories of nominal variables. As an example, consider the variable "political party membership." For this variable, a person may be classified as Democrat, Republican, or Libertarian. That is, a person is not *scored* on political party—he or she simply can be *categorized* into one of the political parties. Also, the coding scheme for data entry could assign a 1 for Democrats, 2 for Republicans, and 3 for Libertarians. Or the code could be 1 for Republicans, 2 for

Libertarians, and 3 for Democrats. Thus, no underlying order with this variable. Collecting these types of information allow to make comparisons between groups, a topic discussed in r the Appendix.

In comparison to other levels of measurement, nominal data are considered to contain the least amount of information. Summarizing nominal data often involves reporting frequencies and percentages.

Ordinal Data

Ordinal data contain slightly more information than nominal level data because the data are ordered, but the space between points on the scale is not equal. Throughout this text, a variety of response scales have been discussed. Consider a 4-point agreement response scale that includes "Strongly disagree," "Disagree," "Agree," and "Strongly agree." If we consider the coding of the data, we might assign 1 for "Strongly disagree," 2 for "Disagree," 3 for "Agree," and 4 for "Strongly agree." The underlying order of the data prevents us from assigning 2 for "Strongly disagree," 4 for "Disagree," 1 for "Agree," and 3 for "Strongly agree." Contrast this ordering of the data with the political example presented earlier. In the instance of the agreement response scale, an underlying order exists, whereas, for the political variable, no underlying order is assumed.

Based on a respondent's choice on an agreement response scale, a researcher would be able to determine generally where the survey respondent fell on the ordered scale. Clearly, one who reports strongly agreeing with a statement has a more positive perception than someone who reports disagreeing. This illustrates the ordered nature of ordinal data. Yet, the difference in perceptions between agreeing and strongly agreeing is not necessarily the same as the difference in perceptions between agreeing and disagreeing. That is, the intervals between the item response options do not reflect the same degree of differences in perceptions.

Ranked data also illustrate the nature of ordinal data. If participants in a professional development program were asked to rank learning modules from least to most relevant, the ranks would represent ordinal (i.e., ordered) data. With this information, an evaluator would be able to determine which module was perceived as being the most relevant to participants. However, the amount of relevance between the modules ranked #1 and #2 might be different from the amount of relevance separating the rankings of #2 and #3. Because the intervals between the points on the item response scale are not equal, mathematical operations are most technically limited to frequencies, medians, and correlations. That said, multiple scholars have demonstrated that ordinal data often behave similarly to interval data (discussed next), which allows for mathematical operations to be performed (Box, 1953, 1954; Hsu & Feldt, 1969; Lunney, 1970). Interested readers should see Lord (1953) for a short account of what convinced "Professor X" that he could compute certain descriptive statistics from ordinal data without needing to lock his door so that students would not see (p. 751).

Interval Data

Data that are ordered and have equal intervals between the data points are classified as interval-level data. Interval data do not have a meaningful zero on the scale, which has important implications for interpretation. **Scale scores** on standardized achievement tests provide an example of interval-level scales. The **raw scores** on standardized tests are often transformed to have a new scale, such as SAT scores being reported on a scale from 200 to 800. Scales might include a value of 0; however, such a score is unlikely to indicate a complete absence of achievement. Therefore, in this instance, the score of 0 is not a meaningful or an absolute zero. Despite not having an absolute zero, interval-level data can be used in mathematical operations. In social science research, the concept of a meaningful zero is often irrelevant. Scores on achievement tests and attitude scales are often treated as if they are at the interval level.

Ratio Data

The level of measurement that contains the most information is ratio, which has order, equal intervals, and a meaningful zero. General examples of ratio-level data are money, height, or weight. A ladder that is 7 feet tall is twice as tall as one that is 3.5 feet tall. This type of relative comparison is made possible by having a meaningful zero. Examples of ratio-level data that may be collected using surveys include certain demographic or personal characteristic variables, such as age in years, or frequency questions, such as the number of professional development modules completed or amount of time a patient spends exercising every day in minutes. Ratio-level data can be subjected to mathematical operations given the equal intervals between points on the metric. Although these kinds of information are not measured using survey response scales, these types of questions are frequently included in surveys and questionnaires to allow studies of the relationship between demographic or personal characteristic variables and the phenomenon of interest as measured by the survey scale.

The four levels of measurement we have described are presented in order of the amount of information each possesses, where nominal data contain the least amount of information and ratio data contain the most. It should be noted that data at the higher, or more information-laden, levels can be transformed into other, lower levels of measurement. For example, if a researcher has the exact ages of her participants, then she can classify them into age ranges, such as 17 or younger, 18 to 25, 26 to 30. Notice that the reverse is not possible. If a different researcher only has the age-range information, then he or she is unable to know the specific age of each participant. Thus, the research or evaluation questions, along with implications for analysis should be carefully considered when selecting the measurement level of input data from survey respondents.

Frequencies

The first type of information many survey developers want to view is the frequency distribution of the responses to their survey. This information will reveal whether the survey participants are using all of the response scales on each item. A frequency distribution is displayed in a table that contains a column with the values present in a set of scores and another column that shows the number of instances, or frequency, for each value in the set. An example of a frequency distribution that might report data from a Likert-type item is shown in Table 7.1. The first column shows all of the values present in a set of responses to a 4-point agreement response scale (i.e., 1, 2, 3, and 4). The second column shows the frequency of each response. Based on this information, one now knows that the 10 responses are 1, 1, 2, 2, 2, 3, 3, 3, 3, and 4.

A frequency distribution can be helpful in diagnosing data entry errors, aiding in determining certain measures of central tendency (i.e., the mode and median), and allowing initial insights into how varied the data are. Suppose the researcher in the scenario described at the beginning of the chapter generated a frequency distribution for all 5,000 students on the first item of the student survey. The response scale contains only four points (i.e., 1, 2, 3, and 4). The hypothetical frequency distribution the researcher generated is presented in Table 7.2.

The frequency table in Table 7.2 shows that 1,351 students selected option 1, 590 students selected option 2, 1,301 students selected 3, and 1,756 students selected option 4. Clearly, there is a problem because the

TABLE 7.1. Frequency Distribution for 10 Student Responses

Response	Frequency	%
1	2	20
2	3	30
3	4	40
4	1	10

TABLE 7.2. Frequency Distribution for 5,000 Student Responses

Response	Frequency	%
1	1,351	27.0
2	590	11.8
3	1,301	26.0
4	1,756	35.1
7	2	0.0

item response scale does not include "7." As a result of this discovery, the researcher can reexamine the dataset to see why this problem occurred. Such troubleshooting is an essential aspect of research and protects the credibility of the instrument and your study. After the problem has been resolved, the frequency distribution can be generated again to show the correct distribution of responses.

Measures of Central Tendency

Measures of central tendency are among the most commonly reported statistics because they summarize much information about a set of data in a single number. In this section, we present three common measures of central tendency: mode, median, and mean.

Mode

The mode is the most frequent data point or value associated with a given variable. It can be used with data collected at all four levels of measurement. Suppose 10 responses to a survey item were selected at random. The item used a 4-point agreement scale, where Strongly disagree = 1, Disagree = 2, Agree = 3, and Strongly agree = 4. The scores in order are 1, 1, 2, 2, 2, 3, 3, 3, 3, and 4. The mode of these scores would be 3 because it is the most frequently occurring value in the string of responses. In data such as these 10 responses, the calculation of the mode is straightforward; however, it is possible to find two or more modes in a set of scores. If two values occur the same number of times and more frequently than all other values, the distribution could be described as bimodal because there are two modes. Sets of scores with more than two modes are multimodal. When every value occurs the same number of times, each value is the mode. It is often helpful to use a frequency distribution as discussed earlier when finding the mode. For example, the distribution of responses from the 5,000 students shown in Table 7.2 has a mode of 4 because 4 was the most frequently reported value.

Median

The median of a distribution is the value that separates scores into the upper 50% of scores and lower 50% of scores. Stated another way, the median is the middle value in an ordered set of values. To find the median of a distribution with an odd number of values, you need only to order the values from smallest to largest and find the value in the middle. When a set of scores has an even number of values, there will be two values in the middle, such as with the 10 randomly selected student responses. Recall that the scores in order are 1, 1, 2, 2, 2, 3, 3, 3, 3, and 4. The values in the fifth and sixth positions are the two middle values, 2 and 3, respectively. To obtain the median of these variables, add the two middle values and divide the sum by two. Thus, the median of the 10 responses is 2.5; that is, $(2 + 3)/2 = 5/2 = 2.5$.

One positive characteristic of the median is that it is not influenced by extreme values, which is why it is commonly used when reporting such demographics as average incomes and body mass index (Penman & Johnson, 2006). In scores with or without extreme values, the median will not change because it does not use all of the data points available. Instead, it only uses the value or values at the center of the distribution. Although using only one or two values is considered a positive aspect of the median in the presence of extreme values, it may be viewed as a negative aspect when no extreme values are present. The median may be used for data measured at the ordinal, interval, or ratio level.

Mean

The mean most often refers to the arithmetic mean and is the most frequently used measure of central tendency. To calculate the mean, all data points are added together and then divided by the number of data points. The mean produces the typical value of a set of scores. To illustrate using the 10 randomly selected scores, the researcher would first need to sum all of the responses: $1 + 1 + 2 + 2 + 2 + 3 + 3 + 3 + 3 + 4 = 24$. Next, this sum is divided by the number of responses: $24 / 10 = 2.4$. Thus, the mean of the 10 randomly selected scores is 2.4.

The mean may be computed for ordinal, interval, or ratio data. Unlike the mode and median, the mean uses all of the data points available in its calculation, which suggests it contains more information. However, when extreme values are present, the mean can be heavily influenced by the extreme values and will become biased. That is, the mean will not necessarily reflect the typical value because it is being more heavily influenced by extreme values that are less representative of the sample as a whole.

Measures of Variability

Measures of variability also provide important information regarding a set of responses because they indicate how similar or different the data are. In this section, we present the range, variance, and standard deviation.

Range

The range is a rather simple measure of variability to calculate in that it reflects the difference between the smallest and largest values in the set of scores. In the set of 10 randomly selected responses, the smallest value is 1 and the largest is 4. Thus, the range for these responses is $4 - 1 = 3$. When do you report the range? If the range for an item that asks students about the quality of their education is 1 on the 4-point scale, then the survey developers know the students tend to have similar perceptions as a group. If they also know the mean is 3.8 ("Strongly agree"), then they know students tend to have positive perceptions about the quality of their education. The survey developers also know that the item does not discriminate between students and their perceptions about the quality of their education. If the item results accurately reflect student perceptions, then the "clumping" of ratings at one end of the response scale is reasonable. In survey development, the range and mean inform the survey developer about the limited use of the response scale.

Variance

The variance is by definition the mean of the squared deviation scores where a deviation score is the difference between a single score and the mean for a distribution. To calculate the variance, one must

1. subtract the mean from every data point (i.e., score),
2. square each difference,
3. add all of the squared differences together, and
4. divide the sum by the number of scores minus 1.

See Table 7.3 for an illustration using the scores from the surveys of 10 randomly selected students.

TABLE 7.3. Example of the Calculation of Variance

Student	Score	Mean score	Deviation (score – mean)	Squared deviation
1	1	2.4	−1.4	1.96
2	1	2.4	−1.4	1.96
3	2	2.4	−0.4	0.16
4	2	2.4	−0.4	0.16
5	2	2.4	−0.4	0.16
6	3	2.4	0.6	0.36
7	3	2.4	0.6	0.36
8	3	2.4	0.6	0.36
9	3	2.4	0.6	0.36
10	4	2.4	1.6	2.56
			Sum	8.4
			Variance	0.93

The variance is a commonly used and reported measure of variability, but it can be difficult to interpret because it is in squared units. However, it is necessary to square the deviations in order to make them all positive. To return the measure of variability back to the original metric, as we will see in the next section, you simply take the square root to obtain the standard deviation.

Standard Deviation

The standard deviation is the square root of the variance of a set of scores, and it is the most commonly reported measure of variability. The standard deviation indicates the typical amount of deviation a score has from the mean. One advantage of using the standard deviation is that it is reported using the same metric as the scores. To calculate the standard deviation, one must simply take the square root of the variance. The variance of the 10 randomly selected responses was previously shown to be 0.93. Therefore, the standard deviation of the responses is $\sqrt{0.93}$ = 0.97. This suggests that the typical amount of deviation from the mean is 0.97 point. If the scores are normally distributed, another way to interpret the standard deviation is that most (68%) of the data points fall within ±0.97 point of the mean.

Measures of Association

Measures of association are used to determine whether a relationship exists between variables, or, said another way, whether two variables **correlate**. Conceptually, the correlation is evaluated by examining how the values of two variables change together, or how they **covary**—that is, looking to see how one variable changes as the other variable changes. An illustration involves student social engagement and grades. An example of an item that was written to gauge social engagement is "I care what other students think about me" (Johnson, Davis, Fisher, Johnson, & Somerindyke, 2000, p. 64). One might hypothesize that as social engagement increases (i.e., students' respond more positively), then grades will generally increase, too. Therefore, one might conclude that student social engagement and grades are related to each other because they covary, or change together. In order to quantify these relationships, **correlation coefficients** are used (usually denoted with the letter r). Correlation coefficients can take any value from -1 to $+1$ and provide two key pieces of information regarding the nature of the relationship between variables. These pieces are direction and strength.

The sign of the correlation coefficients reflects the direction of the relationship. Negative correlation coefficients indicate that as the values of one variable increase, the values of the other variable decrease. A possible example might be number of hours spent watching TV prior to taking an exam and the exam score. Most likely, those who have spent more hours watching TV will score lower on the exam than those who watched less TV. Thus, a negative correlation exists between hours spent watching TV and exam score in this example. Negative correlations are also called indirect or inverse relationships. In the development of a survey scale, we do not typically expect negative correlations. However, on occasion, an item will correlate negatively with other survey scale items and with respondents' total scores. These negative relationships signal the survey developer that the item with a negative correlation might require revision or deletion. We discuss this issue further in Chapter 8.

Positive correlation coefficients indicate that as the values of one variable increase, the values of the other variable increase also. The example using student social engagement and grades illustrates a positive correlation. Positive correlations are also referred to as direct relationships.

The correlation coefficient also provides information related to the strength of the relationship, which is determined by how far away a coefficient is from zero. A coefficient equal to $+1.0$ or -1.0 indicates that a perfect relationship exists between the two variables. This means that a researcher is able to predict exactly what the value of one variable will be by knowing the value of the other. A coefficient of zero suggests that there is no relationship between the variables. That is, having the values of one variable provides no information about the values of the other. An example of a zero correlation would be height and IQ score. Taller people do not have higher IQ scores than shorter people and vice versa.

Scatterplots

The strength, direction, and shape of the relationship between two variables can be determined by examining a plot containing the values of the variables. The plot is called a **scatterplot**. A scatterplot places the values of one variable on the *x*-axis and the values of the other variable on the *y*-axis. A point is placed at each coordinate such that when all data points are plotted, the researcher is able to determine how strongly the variables are correlated, the direction of the correlation (i.e., positive or negative), and the shape of the relationship (i.e., linear or curvilinear). Examples of scatterplots will help illustrate this point.

On one hand, scatterplots that show no pattern (e.g., the data points form an amoeba-like cluster) indicate that there is little to no relationship between the variables. On the other hand, when the scatterplot shows a very consistent and clear pattern, the variables are strongly correlated. Figure 7.1 shows an example of a scatterplot in which there is no discernible

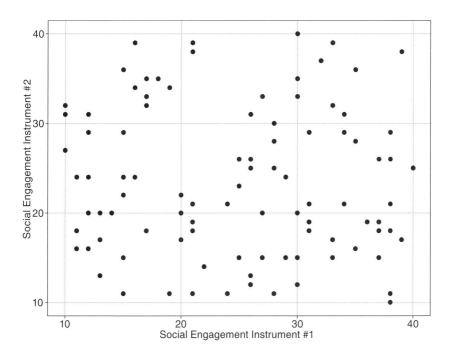

FIGURE 7.1. Example of a scatterplot when two variables demonstrate little to no relationship.

pattern using responses to two social engagement instruments. Each of the two instruments contains 10 items measured with 4-point response scales. If the scores were all added together, the total score for each person would be in the range from 10 to 40. Because of the lack of a correlation, a researcher has no information about a respondent's score on the second social engagement instrument by knowing her or his score on the first social engagement instrument. For example, survey respondents who had a social engagement score of 30 on the first instrument had scores between 12 and 40 on the second engagement scale. The estimate of the Pearson correlation coefficient for the scatterplot in Figure 7.1 is −0.07, which indicates virtually no relationship.

In contrast, Figure 7.2 clearly shows a pattern between the two sets of social engagement scores. By knowing a person's score on the first social engagement instrument, one has a fairly strong indication of the person's score on the second instrument. For example, someone with a score of 30 on the first engagement scale is likely to score in the range of 27 to 33 on the second scale. Thus, there is a strong relationship between the two variables because the values of both variables increase and decrease together (i.e., covary) very consistently across all values. The correlation coefficient

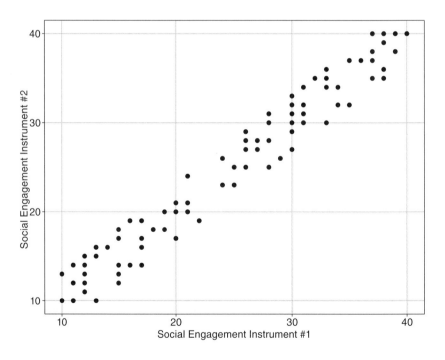

FIGURE 7.2. Example of a scatterplot when two variables demonstrate a strong relationship.

for the variables presented in Figure 7.2 is 0.98. If the two instruments focus on the same aspect(s) of social engagement, Figure 7.2 is closer to the relationship a survey developer might hope to observe between scores on the two instruments.

Recall that for positively correlated variables, as the values of one variable increase so will the values of the other variable. Therefore, the scatterplot should show a positive trend, or a cluster of data points that move from the bottom-left toward the upper-right of the scatterplot. Figure 7.2 illustrates this type of pattern.

A negative correlation coefficient indicates that as one moves up the scale for one variable, she or he moves down the scale on the other variable. A strong, negative relationship between hours spent watching TV the day before the test and percentage of correct test responses is presented in Figure 7.3. Students who spent more time watching television (x-axis) tended to have fewer correct responses on the test (y-axis) and students who spent less time watching television tended to have more correct responses on the test. The correlation coefficient for the variables presented in Figure 7.3 is −0.93.

The remaining characteristic that can be determined with scatterplots is the shape of the relationship. Of primary interest here is whether or not

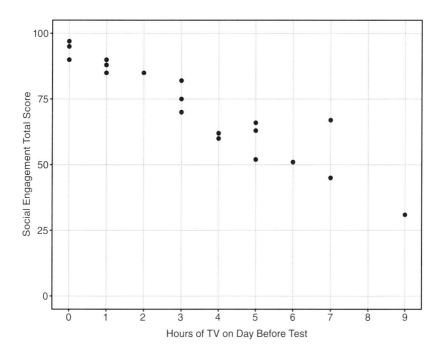

FIGURE 7.3. Scatterplot associated with a strong negative correlation.

the relationship is linear. A linear relationship follows a relatively constant trajectory. That is, for a 1-unit increase in the variable on the x-axis, there is the consistent amount of change in the variable on the y-axis regardless of one's position on X. The scatterplots shown in Figures 7.2 and 7.3 are examples of linear relationships.

A nonlinear relation can take on many forms, such as parabola, hyperbola, or a cubic function. The important point is that the rate of change across values on the y-axis is not the same rate of change for all values on the x-axis. The scatterplot shown in Figure 7.4 shows a nonlinear relationship and exemplifies that the rate and direction of change in Y is not the same for all values of X. Although the correlations presented in this text pertain to linear relationships, it is important for researchers to know when to interpret correlation coefficients. Thus, when the relationship between scores in a scatterplot is not linear, we should not report a correlation.

There are many measures of correlation. Two commonly reported measures of association are the Pearson product–moment correlation coefficient and Spearman's rho correlation coefficient.

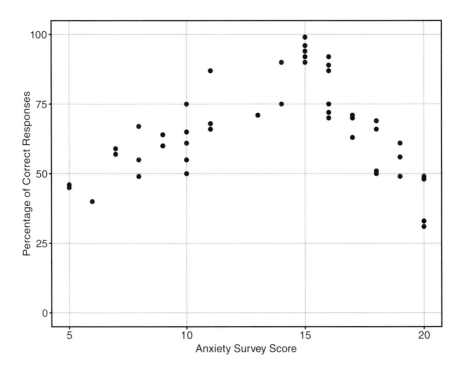

FIGURE 7.4. Scatterplot displaying a nonlinear relationship between scores.

Pearson Correlation

The oft-reported Pearson product–moment correlation coefficient, or Pearson correlation, assumes that the relationship between variables is linear or that the rates of change are constant across the scale. The Pearson correlation should not be used when the relationship between variables is nonlinear. Pearson correlation is appropriate for two interval- or ratio-level variables and is the default correlation coefficient in most statistical software packages.

Spearman's Rho

Another commonly used measure of correlation is Spearman's rho (ρ), which is a correlation coefficient used for ranked or ordinal data. As a result, the Spearman correlation is considered a measure not of linear relationship but rather of monotonic relationship. That is, a researcher interpreting Spearman's ρ can only say that as the values of one variable increase, the values of the other variable either increase or decrease. The researcher is unable to make statements about the rate of change.

Obtaining Descriptive Statistics

Although the measures presented in this chapter can be calculated rather easily, statistical software packages enable users to quickly obtain these descriptive statistics. In this section, the scenario of field-testing a survey for a school district presented at the beginning of the chapter will be used to demonstrate how to analyze data descriptively for both items and scales.

Item Statistics

When analyzing the responses from individual items, the survey developer is probably first interested in some measure of central tendency and variability. In the context of the school district scenario, the survey developer might first review the frequency distributions for each survey item as well as a few descriptive statistics that reflect the general perceptions of all 5,000 students who completed the survey. In SPSS, all of this information can be obtained in one step after the data have been entered.

As shown in Figure 7.5, first click on Analyze from the toolbar and then choose Descriptive Statistics. This will produce a drop-down menu from which Frequencies can be selected.

The Frequencies dialogue box allows users to select which variables they would like to include in the analysis. As shown in Figure 7.6, the first 30 variables are each of the items on the survey. The researcher would highlight the items and move them into the box labeled "Variable(s):."

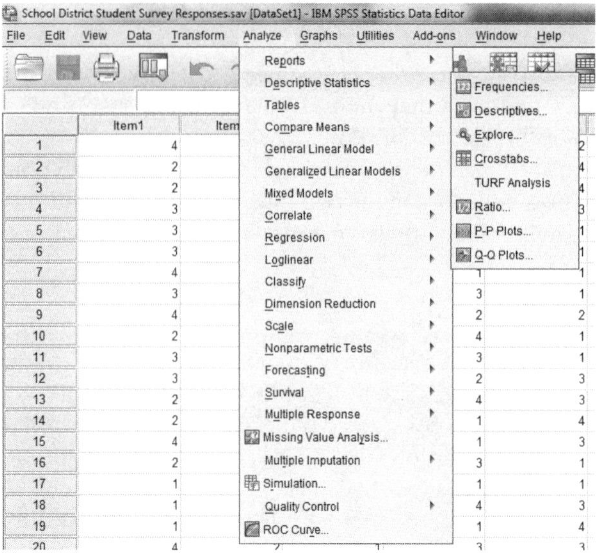

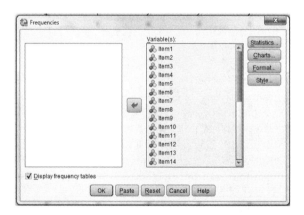

FIGURE 7.5. SPSS drop-down menu from which Frequencies can be selected.

Next, click on the Statistics button to access all of the available statistics that can be calculated using the Frequencies option. The researcher wants to review both the median and mean, which are available under the Central Tendency options, and standard deviation, which is found under Dispersion (see Figure 7.7). From here, click Continue to return to the Frequencies box and then click OK to run the analysis.

FIGURE 7.6. Selection of the items for the analysis.

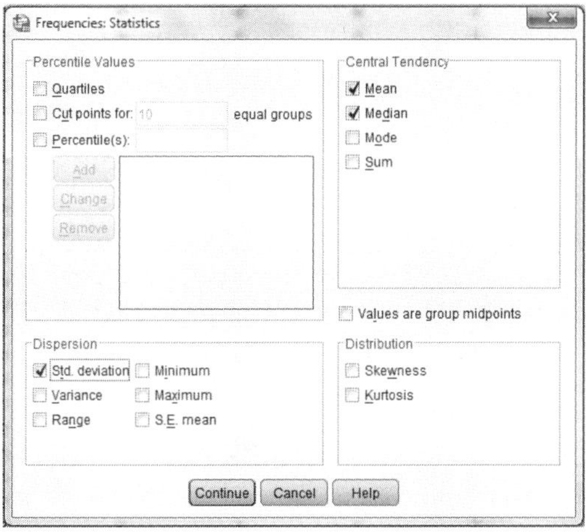

FIGURE 7.7. Selection of the descriptive statistics.

The descriptive statistics for the first five items are presented in Figure 7.8. The first two rows show that the responses from all 5,000 students were used and no data were missing, respectively. The mean for each item is displayed on the third row followed by the median and standard deviation. Based on the means, Item3 had the highest average response at 3.09. This shows that, on average, students rated this item more highly than the other four presented here. Using the medians, one would not be able to discern which item received the highest ratings, on average, in that 50% of the distributions for all five items fall above a rating of 3 and 50% fall below 3. Reviewing the standard deviations, we find that responses to Item3 were also slightly less varied than the other items, though not by much. This reflects that student responses for Item3 tended to be closer to the mean.

Statistics

		Item1	Item2	Item3	Item4	Item5
N	Valid	5000	5000	5000	5000	5000
	Missing	0	0	0	0	0
Mean		2.72	2.84	3.09	2.51	2.65
Median		3.00	3.00	3.00	3.00	3.00
Std. Deviation		1.092	1.068	.938	1.114	1.119

FIGURE 7.8. Descriptive statistics output from the SPSS analysis.

Inter-Item Correlations

To obtain the correlation matrix between the items, first click on <u>A</u>nalyze from the toolbar and then choose <u>C</u>orrelate (see Figure 7.5). This will produce a drop-down menu from which <u>B</u>ivariate can be selected. The Bivariate Correlations dialogue box allows users to select which variables they would like to include in the analysis. The first 30 variables are each of the items on the survey, and Figure 7.9 shows that the first five items have been selected for the analysis. The researcher would highlight the items and move them into the box labeled "Variables:."

The correlations for the first five items are presented in Figure 7.10. The largest estimated correlation coefficient was observed between Item1 and Item2 ($r_{1,2}$ = .115). The weakest estimated correlation coefficient was observed between Item1 and Item4 ($r_{1,4}$ = .002). The letter "N" indicates the number of students who had values for both variables. There were no missing values in the dataset, so all 5,000 students were used in the calculations. The row "Sig. (2-tailed)" refers to statistical significance, a concept developed in the Appendix.

This chapter has explored the use of descriptive statistics to provide information about the specific sample from which data were collected. For

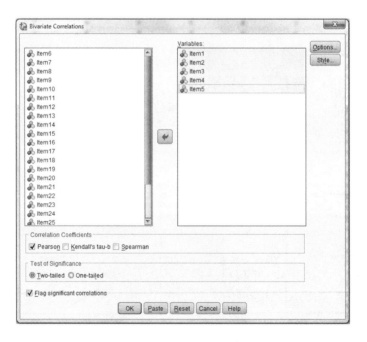

FIGURE 7.9. Items 1 through 5 are selected for correlation analysis.

Correlations

		Item1	Item2	Item3	Item4	Item5
Item1	Pearson Correlation	1	.115**	.080**	.002	.081**
	Sig. (2-tailed)		.000	.000	.888	.000
	N	5000	5000	5000	5000	5000
Item2	Pearson Correlation	.115**	1	.108**	-.003	.073**
	Sig. (2-tailed)	.000		.000	.811	.000
	N	5000	5000	5000	5000	5000
Item3	Pearson Correlation	.080**	.108**	1	.015	.058**
	Sig. (2-tailed)	.000	.000		.286	.000
	N	5000	5000	5000	5000	5000
Item4	Pearson Correlation	.002	-.003	.015	1	.013
	Sig. (2-tailed)	.888	.811	.286		.373
	N	5000	5000	5000	5000	5000
Item5	Pearson Correlation	.081**	.073**	.058**	.013	1
	Sig. (2-tailed)	.000	.000	.000	.373	
	N	5000	5000	5000	5000	5000

**Correlation is significant at the 0.01 level (2 -tailed).

FIGURE 7.10. Correlation output from the SPSS analysis.

the reader interested in making inferences about, or generalizations to, the larger group, we examine the use of parametric inferential statistics in the Appendix. In addition, we discuss the use of nonparametric statistics to analyze survey data that might not meet the requirements for parametric statistics.

In Chapter 8, we apply the descriptive statistics discussed in this chapter to investigate the quality of survey scales. More specifically, we examine item quality, reliability, and validity.

FURTHER READING

Agresti, A., & Finlay, B. (2008). *Statistical methods for the social sciences* (4th ed.). Upper Saddle River, NJ: Prentice Hall.

Provides detailed discussions of descriptive statistics for variables measured at each measurement level. Offers numerous examples.

Kirk, R. E. (2008). *Statistics: An introduction* (5th ed.). Belmont, CA: Thomson.

    Provides detailed discussions of descriptive statistics for variables measured at each measurement level. Offers numerous examples.

Salkind, N. J. (2014). *Statistics for people who (think they) hate statistics* (5th ed.). Thousand Oaks, CA: Sage.

    Discusses descriptive statistics for variables measured at each measurement level. Offers numerous examples. Very readable for beginners.

CHAPTER EXERCISES

1. Identify the appropriate statistics for describing variables measured at the nominal, ordinal, interval, or ratio level.

2. Why can descriptive statistics commonly used for variables measured at nominal level also be applied to variables measured at the ratio level, but not vice versa?

Use the descriptive statistics provided below to answer questions 3 and 4. Each item was measured with a 4-point Likert-type response scale ranging from 1 = "Strongly disagree" to 4 = "Strongly agree."

Descriptive Statistics

	N	Minimum	Maximum	Mean	Std. Deviation
Item10	5000	1	4	3.12	.939
Item11	5000	1	4	3.12	.937
Item12	5000	1	4	2.71	1.109
Item13	5000	1	4	2.68	1.107
Item14	5000	1	4	2.63	1.123
Item15	5000	1	4	3.02	.985
Valid N (listwise)	5000				

3. On which item(s) did respondents tend to report the highest level of agreement?

4. On which item(s) were responses most varied?

Use the correlation matrix provided below to answer Questions 5 and 6.

Correlations

		Item5	Item6	Item7	Item8	Item9
Item5	Pearson Correlation	1				
Item6	Pearson Correlation	.088	1			
Item7	Pearson Correlation	.084	.112	1		
Item8	Pearson Correlation	.111	.099	.099	1	
Item9	Pearson Correlation	.032	.045	.038	.057	1

5. Which two items have the strongest correlation?

6. Which two items have the weakest correlation?

CHAPTER 8

Investigating Scale Quality

The process of validation involves accumulating relevant
evidence to provide a sound scientific basis for the proposed
score interpretations.
—AMERICAN EDUCATIONAL RESEARCH ASSOCIATION,
  AMERICAN PSYCHOLOGICAL ASSOCIATION, AND NATIONAL
  COUNCIL ON MEASUREMENT IN EDUCATION (2014, p. 11)

Introduction

One goal of researchers and program evaluators who use survey scales is to report an accurate score that reflects the extent of a respondent's attitude, the frequency of a behavior, or the depth of knowledge. In this section, we present the types of error that should be controlled and begin a discussion about the concepts of reliability and validity. As shown in Table 8.1, survey results can be influenced by four forms of error: coverage, sampling, nonresponse, and measurement (Leeuw, Hox, & Dillman, 2008).

Coverage Error

Coverage error occurs when some members of a population do not have a chance of being sampled. Such might be the case when a sampling frame (e.g., database or list of the population to be surveyed) has not been updated. The "fix" in this situation is to ensure that the database is current and that all members of the population have a chance of being sampled.

Sampling Error

Sampling error occurs when a subset of members of a population are surveyed. Selection of survey respondents via sampling techniques, such as

TABLE 8.1. Sources of Errors in Surveys

Sources of error	Description	Method for controlling error
Coverage error	When some members of the population have no chance of being selected	Need every member of the population to have a known, nonzero chance of being sampled.
Sampling error	When only a subset of all members of a population are surveyed	Randomly select members of the population and increase the sample size to reduce the error.
Nonresponse error	When some of the sampled members do not respond and differ from those who do in a manner related to the survey	Complete follow-up administrations of the survey for nonrespondents.
Measurement error	When a respondent's score differs from his or her true score	Follow guidelines for item and scale development.

Note. Summarized from Leeuw, Hox, and Dillman (2008).

simple **random sampling** or stratified random sampling, reduces error in survey results. However, any time a researcher surveys a subset of a population, the survey results will contain some error. To reduce sampling error, one can increase the size of the sample or use more precise sampling methods, such as using stratified sampling over simple random sampling. A useful resource on sampling methods is *Sampling in Education and the Social Sciences* (Jaeger, 1984).

Nonresponse Error

Nonresponse error occurs when a large number of a surveyed population does not complete a survey and these nonrespondents differ in a manner related to the survey purpose from those who complete the survey. To reduce nonresponse error, the researcher should complete a follow-up administration of the survey for nonrespondents.

Measurement Error

Measurement error occurs when the respondent's score on a survey scale differs from his or her true score. A respondent's scores might differ from his or her true score owing, in part, to random error, systematic error, or a combination of both. Random error is an issue of reliability, and systematic error is considered an issue of validity (e.g., Streiner, 2003). The collection of evidence about the validity associated with a survey scale is part of the planning, development, and field testing of an instrument. In this chapter, we will describe methods for collecting evidence about the degree to which a survey scale is likely to contribute to valid interpretations of your survey results. We describe procedures for reviewing item and scale quality. Such reviews will provide evidence for the soundness of your proposed score interpretations.

Field Testing

To investigate the quality of a survey scale, prior to administering your operational survey to the targeted respondents, you should conduct a field test. The number of survey respondents in the field test should be large enough to allow statistical analyses to determine if the items and scales have adequate statistical properties. Later in the chapter, we discuss acceptable levels of performance of items and scales.

As we discussed for the pilot test (see Chapter 6), survey respondents in the field test should be similar to those who will complete the planned survey when it is operational. To avoid biasing respondents' answers in the operational survey, the field test should not involve the respondents who will complete the operational survey. Thus, if a patient satisfaction survey will target adults treated in a health care facility, the respondents in a field test should be adults recently receiving health care services from a similar facility. If a research study will involve gathering data about elementary students' attitudes toward reading, then the field test should be conducted with students in a K–5 school that is not part of the study. These field-test participants will provide data that can be analyzed to examine the adequacy of the statistical properties of the items and the validity and reliability associated with the scale.

Response Distributions: Item Quality

To examine item quality, we make use of the descriptive statistics discussed in Chapter 7. These statistics include frequencies, means, standard deviations, and item–total correlations. These qualities inform you about whether the items are functioning appropriately and which items require revision or deletion from the survey.

Frequencies

For Likert-style items a review of the frequencies with which respondents selected each level of an item response scale will be informative. That is, for a 4-point response scale, what percentage of respondents selected 1? What percentage selected 2? What percentage selected 3? What percentage selected 4? Frequencies provide information about whether respondents are using the full response scale. As we discussed in Chapter 5, Dawes (2008) found that the average number of scale points that respondents used for a 5-point response scale was 2.9 (58%), for a 7-point scale 3.6 (51%), and for a 10-point scale 4.0 (40%). So, if respondents arc not using the full item response scale, then a survey developer might consider using a shorter scale or revising the item to elicit more of a continuum of responses.

Why should we be concerned about the distribution of scores across the entire response scale? Recall the previous discussion about the use of survey scales to distinguish between respondents with varied levels of an underlying trait. Thus, we want to distinguish between clients who were satisfied with a service and those who were not. We also want to distinguish between students with positive attitudes toward school and those with less than positive attitudes. If a research study is using a survey scale to place respondents along a continuum for a construct, then the responses should be distributed across the scale. If respondents are not using the full range of the response scale, that is, if a majority of responses are distributed only in the "Disagree" end of the item response scale, or only in the "Agree" end of the scale, then an item does not provide much information that can be used to distinguish between respondents. We revisit here the student engagement item: "I come to school only because my friends are here" (see Table 8.2). A large number of students' responses were in the "Strongly disagree" and "Disagree" categories. Use of the term "only" appears to make the item too extreme. Perhaps the responses would be more evenly distributed if the item under review were edited to state, "I come to school to see my friends."

Frequencies serve another purpose. When data are hand-entered, there is the chance that the responses will be input incorrectly. Completing a frequency analysis allows you to determine whether all the data values are within range for the item response scale or whether any values are out of range. For example, the data for the student engagement scales consisted of values from 1 to 4. Any other value is a miskey. In analysis of the data, most statistical packages provide the option of reporting the minimum and maximum values. The frequency analysis of the items from the Student Engagement Scale provided a minimum value of 1 and a maximum value of 4—consistent with the 1–4 response scale used on the instrument.

A word of caution is important here. If an item is critical to the construct of interest, then discarding the item, or revising the item to the extent that the meaning changes, should not solely occur based on the statistics of the items. Rather, review the wording of the item and examine the frequencies to identify possible changes and submit the problematic item to expert review for recommendations of changing or retaining the item as is.

TABLE 8.2. Frequency Distributions, Means and Standard Deviations, and Corrected Item–Total Correlations for Student Engagement Items

Social engagement items	Strongly disagree[a] N (%)	Disagree N (%)	Agree N (%)	Strongly agree N (%)	Mean (SD)	Corrected item–total correlation[b]
As a ninth-grade student, I . . .						
b. Come to school only because my friends are here.	98 (32.8)	129 (43.1)	43 (14.4)	29 (9.7)	2.01 (0.93)	0.10
c. Care if I finish high school.	4 (1.3)	2 (0.7)	23 (7.7)	270 (90.3)	3.87 (0.46)	0.34
e. Care what teachers think about me.	52 (17.4)	52 (17.4)	109 (36.5)	84 (28.1)	2.76 (1.1)	0.48
h. Often get sent to an administrator for misbehaving.	207 (69.2)	55 (18.4)	23 (7.7)	13 (4.3)	1.47 (0.82)	0.19

Note. N = 299.
[a]Response values were "Strongly disagree" = 1, "Disagree" = 2, "Agree" = 3, and "Strongly agree" = 4.
[b]Corrected item–total correlation is the correlation between an item and the total score after removing the item from the total score.

Mean and Standard Deviation

In the case of Likert-style items, the investigation of item quality is likely to include examination of the mean and standard deviation for each item. The mean and standard deviation also provide useful information about the survey scale and its subscales.

At the item level, the mean and standard deviation provide information about whether respondents used the full response scale. A low item mean, or a very high item mean, indicates responses were at the extremes of the scale. Consider an item response scale of 1 ("Very dissatisfied") to 4 ("Very satisfied"). A mean of 3.8 indicates that a majority of respondents selected the highest response. However, a mean near the center of the response scale is preferable because when responses stack up on one end of the response scale the item might not be worded strongly enough to measure the construct of interest along a continuum (DeVellis, 2012). Returning to the idea that we want a survey scale that locates respondents' status on the scale continuum for the construct, we find that items with extreme means contribute little to differentiating respondents by attitude, by knowledge, or by behavior. In addition, skewed response distributions make it difficult to evaluate relationships with other variables because assumptions for statistical methods are not met.

As discussed in Chapter 7, the standard deviation provides information about the spread of responses around the item mean. The size of a standard deviation is relative to the scale of the item and the spread of the scores. Thus, a 4-point response scale might have a standard deviation of 1.1 as shown in Item e in Table 8.2 or as low as 0.46 as shown in Item c. When all respondents select the same rating, the standard deviation will be 0.

In considering item quality, what standard deviation is desirable? Items with large standard deviations are desirable. A large standard deviation indicates the survey respondents used the full response scale. A small standard deviation (i.e., a standard deviation close to zero) indicates the respondents answered the item similarly, for example, a high majority selecting "Strongly agree." In this case, the survey item fails to place respondents along a scale continuum for the construct.

Total Score

When using scales to assess respondent characteristics, such as attitudes or knowledge, the researcher typically aggregates the study participant's responses to create an overall score. Generally, as the score increases, it is assumed the amount of the construct increases. For example, the intent of the Social Engagement Scale is to sum the scores to obtain an overall score that reflects a student's social engagement. In a study of social engagement and student transition (i.e., passing/failing status), a researcher might investigate the inference that as students' level of social engagement increases, the likelihood of a successful transition (i.e., being promoted) from ninth grade to tenth grade increases.

In some instances, a survey item is negatively worded, as is the item "As a ninth-grade student I often get sent to an administrator for misbehaving" (see Table 8.2). Prior to creating a total score, a researcher will recode this item so that students who respond they "Strongly disagree" with the statement about being sent to the office for misbehaving will receive the highest rating of 4, indicating social engagement. In contrast, a student who responds "Strongly agree" with the statement about being sent to the principal's office will receive the lowest rating of 1, indicating little or no social engagement. With this recoding, the items will aggregate to a high total score for students with high social engagement and a low score for students with low engagement. The total score with recoded data also will be used in calculating the correlation between item responses and total score as well as in estimating reliability and validity coefficients; more on this later.

We do not recommend using recoded data to report frequencies or item means because the meaning of a reverse coded item becomes confusing. Consider Item h in Table 8.2 as an example. As reflected in the frequencies, most of the students either strongly disagreed or disagreed with the statement about often being sent to an administrator for misbehaving. In addition, the item has a low mean ($M = 1.47$). The low mean and high percentage of respondents disagreeing with this item intuitively make sense. We do not expect a majority of students to be sent to the administrator for misbehaving. Thus, recoding is needed for estimation of the correlation between item responses and total score, as well as for reliability and validity coefficients, but not for item means or frequencies.

Corrected Item–Total Correlation

In Chapter 7, we discussed that correlations show how two variables covary. An example of the use of correlations to study whether items covary is the corrected item–total correlation. Also referred to as the item–scale correlation, item remainder coefficient, part–whole coefficient, item–whole coefficient, and the item discrimination index (DeVellis, 2012; Spector, 1992), the corrected item–total correlation quantifies the relationship between an item and the total score for the survey scale after removing the item from the total score. The index ranges from –1.0 to +1.0. Desirable values are above 0.20 (Everitt & Skrondal, 2010). However, for broad constructs, lower correlations might be expected, and for narrowly defined constructs, higher correlations might be expected.

A high corrected item–total correlation indicates that respondents who answered "Disagree" on an item had a low total score and respondents who answered "Agree" on the item had a high total score. For the item on "Care what teachers think about me," the corrected item–total correlation was 0.48, which indicates that students who have a low social engagement total score tended to answer "Disagree" to the statement and students with a high social engagement total score tended to answer "Agree."

In contrast, a corrected item–total correlation of 0.10 for "Come to school only because my friends are here" indicates that students who "disagree" with this item might or might not have a low total score and those who "agree" might or might not have a high total score. Thus, the item does little in helping a researcher to identify students who are socially engaged and those who are socially disengaged. As discussed earlier, the term "only" might have made the statement too extreme. For these reasons, Item b in Table 8.2 would be considered problematic and flagged for further review.

Negative corrected item–total correlations are problematic in that they indicate inconsistency between the responses to an item and the rest of the instrument. That is, respondents who agree with an item tended to have a *low* total score, and those who disagree had a *high* total score. Negative item–total correlations might indicate that an item is negatively worded and not recoded or that an item stem is confusing for respondents.

Revisit Figure 7.3 to see an example of a negative correlation scatterplot. Responses to an item with a negative item–total correlation not only fail to contribute to the measure of a construct, but they might detract from a construct's measurement.

Analyses by Group

Review of items and scales should include analyses by groups. If research studies are likely to include analyses by groups, such as social engagement by gender, then in the field test the items should be reviewed by group. If data from the field test indicate females and males differ on a construct, then changes in one group might mask changes in the overall group. Item analysis by group might assist the survey developer in determining which items are functioning differently for the two groups and in deciding if the items need to be revised or replaced. Given that true differences might exist between groups, statistical methods have been developed to investigate whether there are differences between groups (e.g., females and males) on an item after matching on the level of the construct being measured. Statistical methods for investigating differential item functioning (DIF) allow you to examine statistically whether respondents "with a similar overall ability, or similar status on an appropriate criterion, have, on average, systematically different responses to a particular item" (AERA et al., 2014, p. 16).

Analyses for Knowledge Items

Investigating frequencies, percentages, and corrected item–total correlation is also important for knowledge items. Desirable values for the percentage of respondents who answer an item correctly are in the 50% range. The percentage correct is referred to as a difficulty index.

Desired values for the corrected item–total correlation are 0.20 or higher. In the case of the construct of knowledge, a high corrected item–total correlation indicates that survey respondents with low total scores tended to answer the item incorrectly and respondents with high total scores tended to answer correctly.

Investigating Reliability

Reliability is concerned with the consistency of scores and the various forms of error that contribute to the inconsistency of scores. The review of reliability allows survey developers to examine the consistency of scores associated with a survey scale. When survey scales are used in research, *internal consistency* is often reported (Streiner, 2003; Streiner & Norman,

ypes of Reliability Estimates	
;	Consistency of scores based on . . .
ncy: Cronbach's α	Items within an instrument from a single administration
Coefficient of equivalence/parallel forms	Multiple forms of an instrument with the same distribution of content and item formats, administrative procedures, score means, and standard deviation
Coefficient of stability/test–retest	An instrument administered on different occasions

2008). Less often reported are **score stability** and **parallel forms** (see Table 8.3). In this section, we first discuss the estimation of internal consistency. We then briefly discuss stability and parallel forms of reliability.

Internal Consistency Estimates of Reliability

Internal consistency examines whether the items in the survey scale are a source of error. When selecting items to include on scales, we are sampling from a pool of possible items. An internal consistency analysis provides information about the need to increase the pool of items or remove items that do not fit in the pool. To examine this type of error, survey developers investigate the interrelationships among item responses or scores on separate parts of the survey scale (AERA et al., 2014).

Cronbach's alpha (α) is an often-used measure of internal consistency. Cronbach's α can be used to estimate internal consistency for checklists, for knowledge scales with items scored as right/wrong (e.g., 0, 1), and for Likert-style items. When research involves use of subscale scores and total scores, then α should be calculated for each subscale and the total scale.

Statistical programs such as SPSS, SAS, and R provide Cronbach's α. SPSS has an option for estimation of alpha in the Reliability Analysis window. To navigate to the reliability window, select $\underline{A}$nalyze, then Sc$\underline{a}$le, and then $\underline{R}$eliability Analysis. Select α and the items on your survey scale. SPSS then produces the α coefficient.

Cronbach's α for the Academic Engagement Scale was 0.55, and for the Social Engagement Scale it was 0.56. The internal consistency for the overall Student Engagement Scale was 0.70. One method to increase this α is to increase the number of items in the scale. In *What Is Coefficient Alpha? An Examination of Theory and Applications*, Cortina (1993) illustrated that the number of items has a profound effect on Cronbach's α, especially when correlations between items are low. Also, Duhachek and Iacobucci (2004) illustrated the use of **confidence intervals** to allow readers to better assess the size of the reliability index. Additional forms of internal consistency are discussed in the publications listed at the end of this chapter in "Further Reading."

Coefficient of Stability

Although α coefficient is often reported by survey developers as an estimate of reliability, Cortina (1993) noted that "one must keep in mind the fact that alpha does not offer information about other types of error, such as error associated with stability over time" (p. 102). A coefficient of stability, also referred to as test–retest estimate of reliability, provides information about time or occasions as sources of score error. This measure of consistency is of interest when the survey scale is to be administered to the same respondents on two occasions, perhaps in a test–retest research design. The purpose is to examine whether the change in scores is likely due to measurement error (i.e., occasions). In other words, a single set of survey responses collected at one point in time does not allow a researcher to account for the unique error that may have had an effect only on the single survey administration (i.e., occasion error), but test–retest reliability provides reliability evidence by returning the consistency in responses across multiple occasions.

For example, in a study to improve job satisfaction, researchers want to rule out the random fluctuation of measurement error as contributing to changes in employee attitudes as measured by a job satisfaction scale. Rather, the researchers want to know if change in survey scale scores is due to an intervention and not measurement error associated with the survey scale. Thus, prior to the research study, the research team would field-test the job satisfaction scale. In the field test, on two different occasions survey respondents would complete the scale, and respondents' scores for the two sessions would be correlated. The Pearson correlation can be used for calculation of the stability coefficient (see Chapter 7). A high correlation would mean that the scores have little error due to testing occasions and that any changes in the study participants are likely attributable to the intervention.

This methodology assumes that there is no substantial change in the construct measured between the two occasions. That is, the administration of the survey scale did not cause changes in the apparent preparation of the examinees. Important is the time allowed between the measures. If we measure the same construct twice, the correlation between the two observations will depend, in part, on the amount of time that has elapsed between the two occasions. The shorter the time between the measures, the higher the correlation is likely to be because there is less opportunity for extraneous factors (e.g., unexpected learning) to influence the scores. The stability method of estimating reliability also assumes the respondents have little recall of the actual survey scale items. Thus, this method is likely to overestimate reliability if the items are particularly memorable.

Parallel Forms Reliability Estimates

The parallel forms reliability estimate, also referred to as a coefficient of equivalence, examines whether scores on one form of a survey scale predict scores on another equivalent form of the survey scale. The scatterplot in Figure 7.2 illustrates the consistency of scores across forms (i.e., Form 1 and Form 2).

Researchers use parallel forms of an instrument when the respondents will likely recall items on the scale or for security purposes. So, just as test–retest reliability is used to investigate whether changes in scores are due to occasion error, parallel form reliability provides information about whether changes in scores reflect changes due to the measurement error associated with forms of an instrument. If only one form of a survey is administered, a researcher cannot account for potential error that might result from the specific combination of items (i.e., sampling of items) that appear on the form. The use of a second, parallel form allows the researcher to compare results across forms. If the results are consistent (i.e., strong positive correlation between the responses), then the researcher has some evidence that there might not be error due to the specific items that appear on either form. The parallel forms reliability coefficient also can be calculated using a Pearson correlation.

Evaluating Reliability Estimates

What is an acceptable reliability level? Several sources provide guidance in the interpretation and evaluation of estimates of score reliability. Some authors indicate that research studies and low-stakes assessments require a minimal reliability of 0.70, whereas in applied settings with high stakes, tests generally require a minimal reliability of 0.90 (Herman, Aschbacher, & Winters, 1992; Kaplan & Saccuzzo, 1982; Nunnally, 1978). For research purposes, it is recommended that reliability should be at least 0.70 or higher (Fraenkel & Wallen, 2009), with Streiner and Norman (2008) writing that "internal consistency should exceed 0.8 (p. 9). Phillips (2000) reported that Texas courts found a graduation test sufficiently reliable with total score reliabilities above 0.85.

For research scales, DeVellis (2012) offered the following as acceptable α values:

Below .60—unacceptable
Between .60 and .65—undesirable
Between .65 and .70—minimally acceptable

Between .70 and .80—respectable
Between .80 and .90—very good (p. 109)

He suggested that if α exceeds 0.90, then one should consider reducing the number of items.

The above reliability estimates are based on interpreting individual scores. The evaluation of a reliability estimate also requires consideration of whether interpretation of scores will focus on individual scores or the group mean. For example, Thorndike and Thorndike-Christ (2010) demonstrated that a reliability of 0.70 for individual scores produced stable mean scores for groups composed of 25 members. Hill (2002) demonstrated that a reliability estimate of 0.80 for individual student scores translates to a reliability estimate of 0.87 when based on a group mean composed of 25 members. When making predictions based on a group, Davis (1964) wrote that the reliability coefficient can be as low as 0.50.

Addressing the issue of stability, Streiner and Norman (2008) stated that "it might be reasonable to demand stability measures greater than 0.5. Depending on the use of the test, and the cost of misinterpretation, higher values might be required" (p. 9).

Investigating Validity

The Standards for Educational and Psychological Testing indicate that validity refers to the extent to which evidence and theory support the interpretation of scores for a proposed purpose (AERA et al., 2014). It is not the scale itself that is validated; rather, it is the interpretations and uses of the survey scale scores that are validated (Kane, 2009). The investigation of the validity of interpretations about survey responses proceeds with the collection of forms of validity evidence (see Table 8.4).

Forms of Validity Evidence

What types of validity evidence should one consider when planning a validation study? Forms of evidence to be considered in validating interpretations of scores from survey scales include evidence based on the (1) instrument content, (2) response processes, (3) internal structure, (4) instrument's relationship with other variables, and (5) consequences associated with instrument use (AERA et al., 2014).

Content Evidence

Content validity evidence involves the analysis of the relationship between an instrument's content and the construct it is intended to measure. A

TABLE 8.4. Types of Validity Evidence for Survey Scales

Validity evidence	Purpose of the evidence	Examples of evidence
Content	Review the procedures for specifying the content of the survey scale, the relevance of the content domain to score interpretations, and the degree to which the content of a scale represents the content domain.	Convene a committee of experts to complete a review of survey scale content. Document the review process and outcomes.
Response processes	Identify cognitive processes in which respondents engage when responding to survey items.	Conduct interviews with children to investigate whether their answers are in response to the content of the items or to response options that use smiley-face icons (☹, ☺, ☺).
Internal structure	Examine the extent to which the relationship between survey scale items and scale components (e.g., subscales) align with the construct and the proposed scale interpretations.	Complete a factor analysis to investigate whether the factor structure of the scale is consistent with the construct's theorized structure.
Relations to other variables	Study the extent to which the relationship between survey scale items and other variables (e.g., scales) provide evidence that is consistent with the construct and the proposed scale interpretations.	Correlate scores from a survey scale with scores from another instrument that is intended to measure the same construct.
Consequences	Study the intended and unintended consequences associated with the use of an assessment.	Investigate whether the use of a survey satisfaction scale influences sales staff's focus on customer service.

literature review provides evidence supporting content validity in that the review helps establish the boundaries of the construct domain being operationalized by the survey scale. Demonstrating that the survey items are within the boundaries and representative of the construct domain is one way survey scale developers can provide evidence related to a scale's content validity.

An expert review of the survey scale also provides content validity evidence. For example, in the development of licensure examinations, an organization first completes a job analysis and develops a survey that lists the knowledge, skills, and abilities important to that field (see Figure 8.1). The surveys will be sent to practitioners in the field to provide feedback on the importance of each skill and its frequency. This information, in turn,

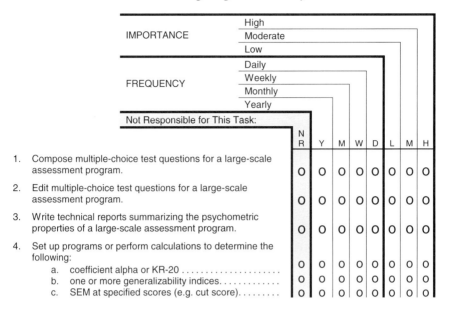

		NR	Y	M	W	D	L	M	H
IMPORTANCE	High / Moderate / Low								
FREQUENCY	Daily / Weekly / Monthly / Yearly								
Not Responsible for This Task:									
1.	Compose multiple-choice test questions for a large-scale assessment program.	O	O	O	O	O	O	O	O
2.	Edit multiple-choice test questions for a large-scale assessment program.	O	O	O	O	O	O	O	O
3.	Write technical reports summarizing the psychometric properties of a large-scale assessment program.	O	O	O	O	O	O	O	O
4.	Set up programs or perform calculations to determine the following:								
	a. coefficient alpha or KR-20	O	O	O	O	O	O	O	O
	b. one or more generalizability indices.	O	O	O	O	O	O	O	O
	c. SEM at specified scores (e.g. cut score).	O	O	O	O	O	O	O	O

FIGURE 8.1. Simulation of a segment of a survey used in a job analysis. From Raymond (2005). Copyright © 2005 John Wiley & Sons, Inc. Reprinted by permission.

will be used to develop the licensure or certification examination. Crocker (2001, p. 2703) outlined the following steps in the content review process:

1. Specifying the questions to be addressed.
2. Defining the domain of interest.
3. Identifying the features of the exercises to be examined in the judgment process.
4. Developing a structured framework for the review process.
5. Selecting qualified experts for that domain.
6. Instructing the experts in the review process.
7. Collecting and summarizing the data.

Typically, when we consider content, we are referring to the items in the instrument and the content those items cover. However, in considering content, the Standards (AERA et al., 2014) included the themes associated with items; the wording and formatting of items; and the guidelines for administration and scoring.

Review of the content domain by a panel of diverse experts might identify sources of irrelevant difficulty (AERA et al., 2014, p. 15). For example, the items on a breast cancer survey scale would be reviewed by a committee of subject matter experts to ensure the appropriateness of items selected to be on the scale for a research study. Items with obscure medical terms that introduce irrelevant difficulty would be rewritten or deleted.

Just as irrelevant difficulty should be addressed in a content review, consideration should be given to identifying bias in representation of groups to remove any stereotypical portrayals. Stereotyping occurs when the language and graphics in materials generalize about people on the basis of irrelevant characteristics, such as physical appearance, dress, or activities (Macmillan/McGraw-Hill, 1993). Bias reviews should attend to the accurate representation of groups by abilities (e.g., physically disabled, gifted, average, mentally handicapped), age, ethnicity, family structure, geographic location, profession, religion, setting (e.g., urban, suburban, rural), sex, sexual orientation, and socioeconomic status. The task of reviewing a survey for stereotypical representation can be made more concrete by considering portrayals of a group in activities, behaviors, dress, environment, language, and physical appearance.

Response Processes Evidence

Investigation of the validity of interpretations also involves examining the fit between the construct and the nature of the performance or response. Validity evidence based on response processes is often based on analyses of individual responses (AERA et al., 2014, p. 15). For example, in a pilot test of an instrument, a respondent could be asked to "think aloud" (Fowler, 2014) or to verbalize his or her thinking about survey scale items.

An example of the use of feedback to gauge responses to survey items comes from a survey scale about ethics and classroom assessment. Figure 8.2 presents two versions of an item related to ethics and classroom

⃠ NOT THIS		
An accounting teacher gives a student an F for the course because the student missed the final exam.	**Ethical** ○	**Unethical** ○
✓ BUT THIS		
An accounting teacher gives a student with a B average an F for the course because the student missed the final exam.	**Ethical** ○	**Unethical** ○

FIGURE 8.2. Example of revision of an item based on response processes.

assessment. Feedback from respondents about the first version of the item indicated that they experienced difficulty in judging the extremity of the teacher's decision in giving a final grade of F because they did not know the student's current grade. The revision to the item added that the student had a current grade of B in order to focus respondents' attention on the teacher's decision to use a grade to punish the student.

Questions about differences in the interpretation of scores between subgroups can be informed by a review of response processes for subgroups (e.g., males and females, African American and white students). Think-alouds or interviews can identify irrelevant or ancillary capabilities (e.g., reading demands in a mathematics test) that are influencing respondents' answers (AERA et al., 2014, p. 15).

FORMS OF RESPONSE BIAS

Response bias is another source of error that potentially interferes with the interpretation of survey results (see Table 8.5). Studies of response bias inform us about whether survey participants' responses are related to the content of the scale or whether their responses are influenced by other cognitive processes. In the instance of response bias, survey participants display a systematic tendency to respond to a range of items on a survey scale on some basis other than the specific item content (Paulhus, 1991). The bias introduces systematic error to the survey results (Schuman & Presser, 1996; Van Vaerenbergh & Thomas, 2013; Villar, 2008), and the introduction of this error undermines the validity of score interpretation (Messick, 1991).

Villar (2008) provided a useful analogy for understanding systematic error. She stated, "The effect is analogous to that of collecting height data with a ruler that consistently adds (or subtracts) an inch to the observed units. The final outcome is an overestimation (or underestimation) of the true population parameter" (p. 751). Thus, the systematic error introduced by forms of response bias possibly will inflate (or deflate) the mean for survey items. In this section, we describe some of the more prominent response biases discussed in the literature, consider when a response bias might be evident, and suggest some methods to lessen the effect of a response bias.

Acquiescence. An **acquiescence** response bias occurs when a respondent displays a tendency to agree with statements regardless of their content (Holbrook, 2008; Schuman & Presser, 1996). Likert-type scales ("Agree"/"Disagree") and true–false items are susceptible to this form of bias. To investigate acquiescence for Likert-type items, a subset of items can be written in positive and negative forms to determine if a respondent

TABLE 8.5. Types of Response Bias

Type	Description: Respondents tend to . . .	When an issue	Methods for reducing bias
Acquiescence	accept or agree with statements regardless of content	Likert scales True–false items Cognitively demanding surveys	Write items in positive and negative forms.
Centrality	use the middle response category of a rating scale regardless of content	Likert-style items	Use an even-numbered scale.
Order effect	allow their answers to earlier survey questions to influence their responses to later questions	Self-administered questionnaire	Use web-based surveys that do not allow respondents to review previous items.
Primacy effect	select options presented first for a visual, self-administered instrument	Self-administered questionnaire	Vary response order in the survey.
Recency effect	select options presented last in an interview	Telephone interviews	Vary response order in the survey.
Social desirability	respond to items in a culturally acceptable direction rather than according to their true feelings	Socially sensitive items	Allow responses to be anonymous. Use self-administered instruments, such as a web survey.

Note. Based on Colton and Covert (2007); Fowler (2014); Messick (1991); Nardi (2003); Oppenheim (1992); Peer and Gamliel (2011); Sax (with Newton, 1997); Schuman and Presser (1996); Schwarz, Knäuper, Oyserman, and Stich (2008); Spector (1992); Thorndike and Thorndike-Christ (2010); Van Vaerenbergh and Thomas (2013); Villar (2008); and Winter (2010).

agrees with both the negative and positive form of a statement. Consider the following:

I care if I finish high school.

Graduating high school is not important to me.

A student who responds "Strongly agree" to both items might be exhibiting an acquiescence response bias. Van Vaerenbergh and Thomas (2013) reported that acquiescence increases with cognitive load. Thus, to lessen acquiescence, survey developers should control cognitive load by wording survey questions clearly and attending to the demands of vocabulary and the length of items.

Centrality. A centrality effect occurs when respondents display a tendency to use the middle response category of a rating scale, regardless of content (e.g., Van Vaerenbergh & Thomas, 2013). This form of response bias is an issue with Likert-style items that use odd-numbered scales. To control for this form of bias, consider the use of an even-numbered scale.

Order. Survey participants' responses display an order effect when initial questions influence their responses to later questions (Peer & Gamliel, 2011). This effect is seen in self-administered surveys that allow survey participants to revisit items and web-based surveys that permit scrolling back to prior questions. A possible method for controlling this form of response bias is the use of web-based surveys that present one item at a time and that do not allow respondents to scroll back to review their responses to previous items.

Primacy. A **primacy effect** occurs when respondents tend to select options presented first in a visual presentation of items (e.g., Schwarz, Knäuper, Oyserman, & Stich, 2008). Thus, this effect may influence survey participants' responses to a self-administered instrument. To avoid a primacy response bias, the order of the response options can be varied in the survey items.

Recency. A **recency effect** occurs when respondents show a tendency to choose the last response options presented to them when the survey is conducted orally (e.g., Schwarz et al., 2008). This form of bias might influence responses from interviews. The effect of a recency response bias may be reduced by varying the response order.

Social Desirability. Desirability response bias refers to a survey participant's tendency to answer items in a culturally acceptable direction rather than according to their actual attitude or feelings (Spector, 1992). To reduce social desirability response bias, Paulhus (1991) suggested that the researcher should assure respondents that their answers are anonymous. In classroom settings, students' perceived anonymity was increased by separating respondents who were friends, indicating that students should not provide identifying marks on the survey, and telling respondents to seal the completed questionnaire in an envelope and drop it in a box as they leave (Becker, 1976; Paulhus, 1991). In a review of forms of response bias, Paulhus noted that previous studies had shown mail surveys to be less susceptible to social desirability response bias. He reported that computerized assessments showed lower social desirability response bias than face-to-face interviews. In contrast, computerized assessments demonstrated higher social desirability response bias than paper-and-pencil assessments. Thus, allowing responses to be anonymous appears to lessen the effect of social desirability.

Internal Structure Evidence

Validity evidence based on internal structure examines the extent to which the relationships among survey scale items and scale components conform to the construct on which the proposed scale score interpretations are based (AERA et al., 2014). One might ask, "Does the construct for an attitude scale specify a single domain, or does it identify several components that are related but are also distinct from one another?" An example is the construct of student engagement. This construct is depicted as consisting of two domains: social and academic. Each brings a unique focus to the construct; however, together they provide information about student's engagement overall. Methods to investigate whether the internal structure of a scale is congruent with dimensions for a construct include factor analysis (see Chapter 9) and multidimensional scaling (Sireci, 2009).

Also, relevant is whether the items function the same for subgroups of respondents. To return to the example of the Student Engagement Scale, do males and females with the same level of social engagement respond similarly across social engagement items? As we described earlier, statistical methods have been developed to investigate whether differential item functioning occurs for respondents after matching on the level of the construct being measured. That is, do respondents with a similar overall ability (e.g., social engagement scores), have systematically different responses to a particular item (AERA et al., 2014, p. 16)? Although a discussion of DIF is beyond the scope of this book, interested readers will find useful the resources listed in the "Further Reading" section at the end of this chapter.

Relations to Other Variables

Validity arguments frequently include evidence about the relation of instrument scores to measures external to the instrument. Of interest is the degree to which the relationships are consistent with the proposed interpretations associated with the construct. Investigations include studies of instrument–criterion relationships and convergent and discriminant evidence.

INSTRUMENT–CRITERION RELATIONSHIPS

Criterion-related validity evidence expresses the association between scores on the scale and scores associated with a defined outcome. Two forms of criterion-related validity evidence are concurrent validity evidence and predictive validity evidence.

Concurrent validity evidence provides information about the association between a survey scale and an alternative instrument of the same construct (AERA et al., 2014). Respondents' scores on a survey scale and an alternative scale are collected concurrently. To examine concurrent validity for the Student Engagement Scale (SES), student scores could be correlated with the relevant scores from the Academic Competence Evaluation Scales (ACES; DiPerna & Elliott, 1999, 2000). The ACES includes scales that measure students' Interpersonal Skills, Academic Motivation, and Study Skills. These scales appear to gauge student social engagement and academic engagement and could provide concurrent validity evidence. That is, both the SES and ACES could be administered to a group of examinees, total scores calculated for each instrument for each respondent, and the totals correlated to examine if these two instruments are measuring the same construct.

Predictive validity evidence provides information about whether a score on a survey scale predicts future behaviors, such as the purchasing decisions of consumers. A student engagement scale might be studied to determine if it predicts student promotion or student high school graduation.

CONVERGENT AND DISCRIMINANT VALIDITY EVIDENCE

Validity studies include the collection of convergent and discriminant evidence to investigate the appropriateness of interpretations and uses of the data (Messick, 1993). In collection of convergent validity evidence, we examine whether two measures that we expect to be related are actually related in an empirically demonstrable manner. In one form of this type of validity evidence, "criterion groups are identified that are expected to differ with respect to the construct being measured" (Messick, 1993, p. 55). The Student Engagement Scale provides an example of two groups that differ with respect to academic engagement. The students earning a pass or a fail for their English class formed the criterion groups. On a 4-point scale, the student mean for the item "As a ninth-grade student I complete all my work" was 3.07 for passing students and 2.67 for failing students. For the item "As a ninth-grade student I study to prepare for tests," the mean was 3.09 for passing students and 2.42 for failing students. Not all items performed as expected. For the item "As a ninth-grade student I come to class without books, pencil, or paper," the mean was 1.84 for passing students and 1.70 for failing students. Thus, the comparison of criterion groups provided some evidence of convergent validity.

To study discriminant validity, the survey scale developer collects evidence about two measures that are *not* expected to be related. She examines whether the measures are actually not related in an empirically demonstrable manner. For example, in a math word problem test, scores from this assessment and a verbal test could be correlated to determine the extent to which verbal ability influences math scores (i.e., introducing construct irrelevant variance to scores).

High correlations between assessments indicate that the measures appear to converge on a construct. Student engagement scores, for example, might correlate with the number of school activities in which students' participate, thus converging on the construct of engagement. Discriminant evidence, such as low correlations between student engagement scores and student socioeconomic status, would indicate that the survey results are not related to extraneous constructs. Taken together, convergent and discriminant evidence provide information about the appropriateness or validity of inferences (Messick, 1993).

Evidence Based on the Consequences of Testing

Validity evidence related to the consequences of testing refers to the evaluation of the intended and unintended consequences associated with use of an assessment. In education, this evaluation includes adverse impact, the influence of testing on instruction, and the influence of testing on dropout rates (Sireci, 2009).

In Chapter 2, we stated that the construction of a survey scale is a demanding process. The process of validation includes defining the construct, stipulating the proposed interpretations from the scores from an instrument, stating a validity argument, identifying relevant validity evidence, collecting the evidence, and integrating that evidence. In this manner, "A sound validity argument integrates various strands of evidence into a coherent account of the degree to which existing evidence and theory support the intended interpretation of test scores for specific uses" (AERA et al., 2014, p. 21).

These numerous aspects of validation can be daunting. To provide guidance in this process, Kane (2001, p. 330) outlined the following steps for validation:

1. State the proposed interpretive argument as clearly and explicitly as possible.

2. Develop a preliminary version of the validity argument by assembling all available evidence relevant to the inferences and assumptions in the interpretive argument. One result of laying out the proposed interpretation in some detail should be the identification of those assumptions that are most problematic (based on critical evaluation of the assumptions, all available evidence, and outside challenges or alternate interpretations).

3. Evaluate (empirically and/or logically) the most problematic assumptions in the interpretive argument. As a result of these evaluations, the interpretive argument may be rejected, or it may be improved by adjusting the interpretation and/or the measurement procedure in order to correct any problems identified.

4. Restate the interpretive argument and the validity argument and repeat Step 3 until all inferences in the interpretive argument are plausible, or the interpretive argument is rejected.

As we discussed earlier, the validation of an instrument benefits from the collection of evidence about the internal structure of the survey scale. In Chapter 9, we discuss factor analysis, which is a procedure that allows a survey developer to examine the relationship between survey items and the internal structure of the data.

FURTHER READING

Camilli, G. (2006). Test fairness. In R. Brennan (Ed.), *Educational measurement* (4th ed., pp. 221–256). Westport, CT: American Council on Education and Praeger Publishers.

> *Provides an in-depth treatment of statistical methods for investigating differential item functioning in items.*

Clauser, B., & Mazor, K. (1998). Using statistical procedures to identify differentially functioning test items. *Educational Measurement: Issues and Practice, 17*(1), 281–294.

> *Introduces the reader to statistical methods for examining differential item functioning in items.*

De Ayala, R. J. (2009). *The theory and practice of item response theory.* New York: Guilford Press.

> *Chapter 12 of text provides in-depth and reader-friendly treatment of DIF.*

Jaeger, R. M. (1984). *Sampling in education and the social sciences.* New York: Longman.

> *Provides an in-depth discussion of sampling methods, estimators, and applications.*

Meyer, J. P. (2010). *Reliability.* New York: Oxford University Press.

> *Provides an in-depth treatment of reliability.*

Salkind, N. (2012). *Tests and measurement for people who (think they) hate tests and measurement.* Thousand Oaks, CA: Sage.

> *Introduces the reader to the concepts of reliability and validity.*

Streiner, D. L. (2003). Starting at the beginning: An introduction to coefficient alpha and internal consistency. *Journal of Personality Assessment, 80*(1), 99–103.

> *Provides a brief introduction to Cronbach's α and internal consistency.*

CHAPTER EXERCISES

1. In Table 8.2, for the item "As a ninth-grade student I care what teachers think about me," which option was selected by the most students? In terms of item quality, is this a desirable value (i.e., percentage)?

2. For the item "As a ninth-grade student I care if I finish high school," what is the corrected item–total correlation? Is this a desirable value?

3. Another item on the Student Engagement Scale asked students to respond to the statement "As a ninth-grade student I have many friends at school." The mean was 3.50. In terms of item quality, is this a desirable scale? Why or why not?

4. In a field test to develop a student engagement scale, the corrected item–total correlation was .611 for the statement "I feel teachers care about me." Would you use this item in a student engagement scale? Support your answer.

5. In preparing to develop items for a job satisfaction scale in home health care, the survey developer completed a literature review to determine the domains that the items should measure. The literature review contributes to what form of validity evidence?

6. A survey developer field-tests a job satisfaction scale with a sample of home health care workers. She also asks the supervisors to assign an overall satisfaction rating for each health care worker. The survey developer then correlates the health care workers' scores and the supervisor's scores. What form of validity evidence is the survey developer studying?

7. The reliability for the job satisfaction scale was 0.85. Is this an acceptable level? Support your answer.

CHAPTER 9

Factor Analysis

Exploratory factor analysis is not, or should not be, a blind process in which all manner of variables or items are thrown into a factor analytic "grinder" in the expectation that something meaningful will emerge.
—PEDHAZUR AND SCHMELKIN (1991, p. 591)

Introduction

In the previous chapter, we discussed how factor analysis can provide evidence for the validation of a survey scale. Specifically, we presented factor analysis as a procedure that provides information about the internal structure of the instrument. In this chapter, we provide greater detail about conducting a factor analysis.

Let's begin our discussion with a thought experiment. Suppose you were given a list that consisted of *dog, computer, fish, guinea pig, cat, cell phone, television*, and *digital camera*, and you were asked to group these things into as many categories as you thought were appropriate. Most likely, you would organize the objects in the list into two categories: pets and electronic devices.

Now consider a set of eight survey items that were all written to measure teachers' views of a professional development program's effectiveness. Such professional development programs are commonly composed of many different aspects, such as leadership, implementation, instructional materials, level of funding, and perceived benefits. Following the item-writing guidelines in Chapter 4, eight items could be written to potentially measure teachers' views of each of these program elements. As we discussed in Chapter 4, it is important to remember that each item should measure only one program element, such as leadership or implementation, but not both in the same item (see Figure 9.1).

143

<table>
<tr><td></td><td colspan="4">⊘ NOT THIS</td></tr>
</table>

	Strongly disagree	Disagree	Agree	Strongly agree
1. The presenter(s) was/were knowledgeable and well prepared.	1	2	3	4

✓ BUT THIS

	Strongly disagree	Disagree	Agree	Strongly agree
1. The presenters were knowledgeable.	1	2	3	4
2. The presenters were well prepared.	1	2	3	4

FIGURE 9.1. An example of addressing only one element in an item.

In Figure 9.2, each row and column represents one of eight items. For illustration purposes, suppose a plus sign ("+") indicates that a relationship exists between those scale items where the row and column intersect. That is, when teachers, for example, assign a high rating to Item 1, they also tend to assign a high rating to Item 2. Teachers who assign a low rating to Item 1 also tend to assign a low rating to Item 2. The table shows that Items 1, 2, 3, and 4 are all related to each other but are not related to any other items. Conversely, Items 5, 6, 7, and 8 are related to each other but are not related to the other items. In other words, Items 1 through 4 appear to have something in common, and Items 5 through 8 appear to have something in

	Item 1	Item 2	Item 3	Item 4	Item 5	Item 6	Item 7	Item 8
Item 1		+	+	+				
Item 2	+		+	+				
Item 3	+	+		+				
Item 4	+	+	+					
Item 5						+	+	+
Item 6					+		+	+
Item 7					+	+		+
Item 8					+	+	+	

FIGURE 9.2. An example of a matrix that depicts the relationship between survey scale items.

common. One might infer in this case that the relationship between Items 1, 2, 3, and 4 indicates that this group of items is assessing one construct, whereas the relationship between Items 5, 6, 7, and 8 indicates that these items are measuring some other construct. Importantly, the lack of a relation between Items 1, 2, 3, 4 with Items 5, 6, 7, and 8 indicates that the items assess two separate constructs. Defining what these two constructs actually are is discussed later in the chapter.

Conceptually, this is the basis of exploratory factor analysis (EFA)— examining relationships between a given set of items to determine the number of constructs that are being measured by the items. When data that were collected using a survey scale are analyzed, the table (i.e., matrix) of item relationships will contain correlation coefficients that are produced by a statistical software package. Correlation coefficients indicate relationships between two variables, as discussed in Chapter 7.

Unfortunately, data collected in real-world research are not likely to be as easily interpreted as presented in the matrix above, but, given the processing speeds of modern personal computers and statistical software packages, using exploratory factor analysis to make sense of complex datasets is well within reach for survey scale developers. Although few patterns similar to the one presented in Figure 9.2 may be evident based on visual inspection, EFA can be carried out using statistical packages to mathematically study the underlying structure (i.e., number of **factors**) of a set of items. In essence, EFA refers to a family of statistical procedures used to provide evidence for the number of constructs (i.e., factors) that are being measured by a collection of measured variables, such as survey scale items.

In Chapter 9, we describe the use of factor analysis to explore the dimensionality of constructs, such as student engagement or job satisfaction of health care workers. Over the course of this chapter, we discuss various components and processes in conducting factor analysis. First, the general purposes and processes of factor-analytic procedures will be described. Second, we discuss the viability of factor solutions being contingent on the tenability of underlying assumptions. Third, we address the importance of understanding the underlying dimensional structure of a dataset. Fourth, **principal axis factoring** is described, including considerations and implications for its use. Fifth, the common procedures for determining the number of factors are presented. Sixth, rotation methods are introduced, and several examples are presented and explained. Finally, guidelines for interpreting factor-analytic solutions are provided. Sample output from IBM SPSS Statistics software (SPSS)[1] with annotations are included throughout the chapter.

---

[1]SPSS® Inc. was acquired by IBM® in 2009. IBM, the IBM logo, *ibm.com*, and SPSS are registered trademarks of International Business Machines Corporation.

General Purposes and Processes
Associated with Factor-Analytic Procedures

Sheskin (2007) wrote that a complex set of mathematical operations is required in order to factor-analyze a matrix (i.e., table) of item correlations. Fortunately for researchers, the algorithms for the various factor-analytic procedures have been programmed into many of the statistical software packages, and thus, underlying mathematical operations will not be discussed in this text. In essence, the statistical algorithms analyze the correlation matrix to assist researchers in determining whether the set of items can be reduced to a smaller number of **latent variables** (Sheskin, 2007), or constructs. Before conducting a factor analysis, one must, of course, hypothesize that constructs *actually* underlie the dataset. In other words, the construct(s) is/are hypothesized to influence the responses to items. The focus then is to separate the total variance (i.e., variability) in the item responses into the variance that is shared between items, the variance that is unique to each item, and the variance that is due to error. Andrews (1984) described this as partitioning the total variance into "valid variance," "correlated error variance," and "random error variance" (p. 410). Correlated error variances are related to method effects, which is a type of measurement error that we discussed in Chapter 8. In his review of five national surveys, Andrews reported that between 50 and 83% of the total variability in survey responses could be explained by the valid variance (i.e., construct of interest), between 0 and 7% of the total variability could be explained by the method effect variance, and between 14 and 48% of the total variability could be explained by the error variance. This is an important issue that will be discussed in more depth in the section "Extraction: Principal Axis Factoring."

When examining the relationship between any two survey scale items, it is possible to control for a third variable by mathematically partitioning out its relationship with the two original items. The resulting relationship is called a partial correlation. In essence, the factor-analytic algorithm finds the partial correlations between items controlling for the underlying construct. These partial correlations will be small if there is a strong underlying dimensional structure. In fact, the smaller the partial correlations are, the stronger the influence of the underlying factor.

Testing Assumptions

The viability of factor-analytic solutions is contingent on the tenability of certain underlying assumptions. First, linearity is assumed of all bivariate relationships. This is easily assessed by examining bivariate scatterplots (see the discussion of scatterplots in Chapter 7). The second assumption is the absence of extreme collinearity (i.e., very high correlations) or singularity (i.e., perfect correlation) between items. Extremely collinear items have significant overlap in the information they add to the solution, and singular items provide exactly the same information. Thus, one might consider removing these items from the modeling because they do not add anything statistically unique to the model. Ultimately, the decision to remove items from the modeling should take into account both statistical and substantive information. That is, if extremely collinear items provide unique substantive information, then a survey developer may consider including the items in the model.

Dimensionality

The factor structure of a construct can be **unidimensional** or **multidimensional**. In this section, we discuss the implications of the dimensionality of a construct.

Unidimensionality

With varying levels of awareness, many educators are already familiar with the concept of unidimensionality because it is commonly assumed when developing and scoring tests. On most assessments, students are accustomed to receiving a single score. This is true because it is assumed that there is only one factor influencing test performance—the student's ability in a specific (i.e., unidimensional) content area. Thus, the single score is a representation of the amount of knowledge possessed by the student in that content area.

The number of factors underlying a set of item responses has important implications for analysis and decisions made based on data collected with scales. A scale is said to be unidimensional when the entire set of items measures only one underlying factor. Furr and Bacharach (2009) noted that responses to a unidimensional set of scale items are related to only one attribute and are not affected by a person's other attributes. Of course, a scale is never believed to be completely unidimensional (i.e., 100% of variance is explained by the single underlying factor). Instead, unidimensionality is considered plausible based on the presence of a single "dominant" factor, that is, a single factor that most influences one's responses to a set of items, or a factor that explains most of the variation in responses. When a set of items is determined to reflect the same underlying construct, then scores can be calculated based on the individual item responses that reflect an overall amount or position on the construct.

The diagram in Figure 9.3, called a path diagram, shows how a unidimensional scale can be visualized. Note that the circle represents the single

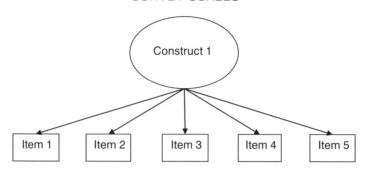

FIGURE 9.3. An example of a set of unidimensional items.

factor and the squares represent five items that comprise the survey scale. The arrows are pointing from the construct to the items because the direction of the arrows indicates that a person's response to each item is due to how much (or little) of the construct the person possesses.

Returning to our previous example, we find that if the construct being measured above was teachers' perceptions of the effectiveness of a professional development program, then the teachers' perceptions would determine how they responded to these eight items. If a person viewed the professional development program as being very effective, then she or he would likely respond very favorably to items about program effectiveness. Therefore, in a path diagram, the arrows, or paths, should be drawn from the construct(s) to the observed variable(s).

Multidimensionality

A set of items that measure more than one construct is said to be multidimensional. Although determining the number of factors will be discussed later in this chapter, it is important first to explore the implications of having multiple constructs underlying a set of item responses. For a multidimensional set of items, the psychometric qualities as discussed in Chapter 8 should be examined for each subset of items (Furr & Bacharach, 2009). Consider once again instances from testing. On tests for admission to undergraduate and graduate programs, scores are given for quantitative and verbal abilities because the two abilities, though possibly related, are considered to be distinctly different constructs. Factor-analytic procedures take into account the inter-item correlations and return information that informs researchers' decisions about the potential number of constructs underlying the set of item responses.

The path diagram in Figure 9.4 shows how a scale with two unrelated factors can be visualized. Construct 1 is shown to be influencing responses to Items 1 through 3, and construct 2 is shown to be influencing Items 4

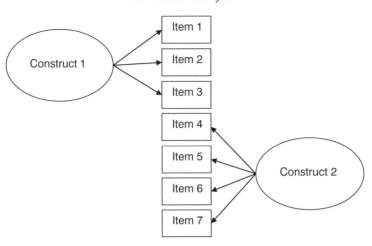

FIGURE 9.4. An example of a set of multidimensional items.

through 7. If the factors are correlated, the path diagram will include a curved two-headed arrow between the factors (see Figure 9.5).

Extraction: Principal Axis Factoring

Extraction generally refers to the method by which factors are identified as underlying a set of responses. There are several extraction methods, but we discuss principal axis factoring (PAF) as it is the most commonly used

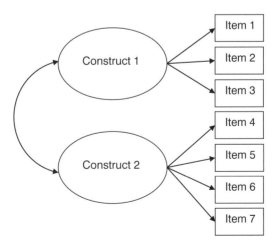

FIGURE 9.5. An example of a path diagram for correlated factors.

extraction method. For a discussion of different extraction methods, see Brown (2006).

PAF is also known as common factor analysis or exploratory factor analysis, or it may be simply referred to as factor analysis. In its calculations, PAF only uses the variation that is shared between items. These shared variations are called communalities, which are in essence the relationship between each item and all other items collectively. The purpose of PAF is to determine the number and nature of factors that underlie the set of responses and account for the shared variation (Hatcher, 1994). Thus, PAF is commonly used for model testing because it only models the shared variation and ignores the variation that is unexplained. PAF requires the estimation of communalities between items, which makes it more mathematically complex, but this issue is mitigated thanks to the processing power of current computers.

The major benefits of PAF extraction are that (1) there are no distributional assumptions and (2) it is always possible to obtain results. A disadvantage of PAF extraction is that no fit statistics are provided to assist the research with model selection. However, there are many other types of evidence that assist with model selection, so the lack of fit statistics is not a major drawback.

Determining the Number of Factors (Model Selection)

After the extraction method is selected, the next step is to determine the number of factors to extract. This is the most crucial decision, and it should be guided by substantive considerations and statistical information. A strong literature review will greatly improve interpretability. In this chapter, we will present several types of information that should be evaluated when determining the number of factors, including the Kaiser criterion (i.e., eigenvalues > 1.0), visual inspection of the **scree plot**, parallel analysis, the reproduced residual matrix, and **factor loadings**. An example will help explain each of these topics. As an illustration, we will use a 14-item instrument designed to measure satisfaction with the various aspects of one's job.

Eigenvalues

Kaiser (1960) proposed that the number of factors to be extracted should be equal to the number of factors with eigenvalues greater than 1.0. An **eigenvalue** is the amount of variation explained by a factor (Widaman, 2007). Sheskin (2007) noted that an eigenvalue is an index that represents the relative strength of each extracted factor. In essence, an eigenvalue reflects the amount of information provided by one item. Therefore, the sum of the eigenvalues in any given model is equal to the total number of items in the model. It makes sense, then, that one would only want to retain factors that explain more variation than a single item. That is, one would only want to retain the factors with eigenvalues greater than 1.0. As seen in the Initial Eigenvalues column of Figure 9.6, the first extracted eigenvalue is 7.444, which accounts for 53.17% of the variance in the set of item responses. The second eigenvalue is 1.635 and explains an additional 11.68% of the variance. All remaining factors have eigenvalues less than 1.0 and therefore account for less variance than a single item. This provides evidence that two factors underlie the dataset. It should also be noted that Fabrigar, Wegener, MacCallum, and Strahan (1999) suggested that factor solutions should explain more than 50% of the total variance.

Total Variance Explained

Factor	Initial Eigenvalues		
	Total	% of Variance	Cumulative %
1	7.444	53.170	53.170
2	1.635	11.681	64.852
3	.873	6.234	71.086
4	.680	4.856	75.942
5	.505	3.604	79.546
6	.470	3.360	82.906
7	.429	3.062	85.968
8	.386	2.758	88.726
9	.345	2.464	91.191
10	.322	2.300	93.490
11	.276	1.974	95.464
12	.249	1.779	97.243
13	.224	1.599	98.842
14	.162	1.158	100.000

Extraction Method: Principal Axis Factoring.

FIGURE 9.6. An example of initial eigenvalues in exploratory factor analysis.

Scree Plot

The second piece of information to consider in selecting a factor solution is the scree plot, first proposed by Cattell (1966), which simply plots the eigenvalues. In addition to looking at the eigenvalue table, one might also look to see where the scree plot levels off or the point at which an elbow appears in the plot. The scree plot for the job satisfaction instrument is presented in Figure 9.7. From Factors 3 to 14 (see arrows in Figure 9.7), the plot seems to be rather smooth, which suggests that there are again only two factors underlying the set of responses. The number of factors to be extracted based on the scree plot is equal to the number of factors *before* the line levels off. In other words, one should count the number of steep drops in order to determine the number of factors to extract. In Figure 9.7, there is a steep drop between Factors 1 and 2 and another relatively steep drop between Factors 2 and 3. Therefore, the scree plot provides evidence that two factors should be extracted. It should be noted that often in practice the scree plot will not have a clearly defined elbow. The researcher should therefore consider all of the pieces of information (i.e., eigenvalues, scree plot) regarding the number of factors to extract and make a decision that is best supported collectively by the information.

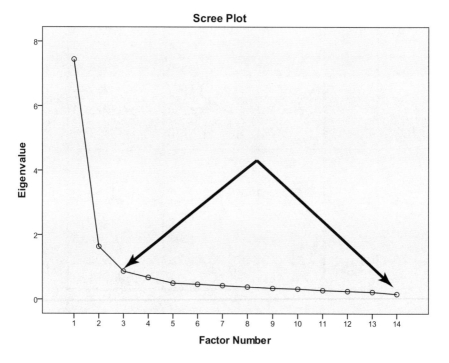

FIGURE 9.7. Sample scree plot.

Parallel Analysis

The third piece of information to consider in selecting a factor solution is the results of parallel analysis, which also uses eigenvalues. In parallel analysis, many datasets are simulated, each of which contains the same number of variables and the same number of respondents. The difference is that each dataset is made up of completely random data. The eigenvalues are computed for each dataset, and the mean is computed across all of the datasets. Table 9.1 shows the results based on 1,000 parallel analyses. The eigenvalues computed from the parallel analysis for the real dataset are compared against the mean eigenvalues from datasets consisting of random numbers. The number of factors indicated by parallel analysis should be the number of eigenvalues that are more extreme than those returned from the random datasets. The first four factors have eigenvalues more extreme than the mean eigenvalues from the randomly generated datasets. Therefore, the four factors should be evaluated according to parallel analysis. Multiple studies have shown that parallel analysis may be useful for determining the correct number of factors (Humphreys & Montanelli, 1975; Zwick & Velicer, 1986), but this may depend on the correlation matrix used in the analysis. Buja and Eyuboglu (1992) noted that parallel analysis may return

TABLE 9.1. Results from Parallel Analysis

Factor	Eigenvalues from real data	Mean eigenvalues from 1,000 datasets of random numbers
1	7.057308	0.355817
2	1.224989	0.277884
3	0.405458	0.217170
4	0.204779	0.165698
5	0.099651	0.120084
6	0.032778	0.077629
7	−0.00383	0.038193
8	−0.02715	−0.00082
9	−0.07195	−0.03932
10	−0.09046	−0.07575
11	−0.10204	−0.11333
12	−0.12184	−0.15237
13	−0.14469	−0.19462
14	−0.17644	−0.24293

too many factors in the case of principal axis factoring as opposed to principal components analysis (see "Further Reading" for more information). Although four eigenvalues were observed beyond pure chance, all evidence should be considered together in determining the number of factors underlying a set of item responses.

Reproduced Residual Matrix

The fourth piece of information to consider in selecting a factor solution is the reproduced residual matrix. Residuals are generally what is left unexplained after a statistical model has accounted for as much variation as it can. In the case of PAF, the model being examined is used to create a new correlation matrix, which is then compared to the original matrix. Next, the difference is taken between the original correlation coefficients and the reproduced correlation coefficients in the hopes that the differences, or residuals, will be very small. The reproduced residual matrix contains all of these differences along with the frequency and percentage of residuals with absolute values greater than 0.05. As seen in the note in Figure 9.8, 19 residuals (20.0%) have absolute values greater than 0.05. Ideally, the reproduced residual matrix would contain fewer than 5% residuals greater than |0.05|, but the factor solution that produces the smallest residuals may also be supportive of a particular factor solution. In order to make these comparisons, multiple models would need to be compared and considered.

Factor Loadings

The factor loadings are the final piece of information to consider for a factor solution. Factor loadings can be interpreted as a type of measure that expresses the strength of the relationship between an item and each factor. In an ideal factor solution, each item will have a high factor loading on one factor and load very weakly on the other factors. Each factor should also have three or more items that load onto it. Such a solution was first described by Thurstone (1947) as having simple structure, which is typically desired for a solution in which items load onto more than one factor.

How large a factor loading must be to indicate a "strong" relationship between the item and factor has long been a topic for debate. Traditionally, a factor loading of 0.4 is used as the lower bound of an acceptable loading. Square correlation coefficients reflect the proportion of variance of one variable explained by another. Thus, a loading of 0.4 indicates that the factor explains 16% ($0.4^2 = 0.16$, or 16%) of the variance in the item responses. More recently, Stevens (2009) posited that factor loadings should use statistical significance tables to determine appropriate levels of strength. In other words, a loading that exceeded a particular critical value for statistical significance was sufficiently strong. Yet, such methods are heavily influenced

Reproduced Correlations

	v1	v2	v3	v4	v5	v6	v7	v8	v9	v10	v11	v12	v13	v14
Residual[b] v1		.036	-.028	.051	-.001	-.024	.029	.018	-.053	-.001	-.023	-.009	.026	-.018
v2	.036		-.010	-.075	-.044	.055	.021	-.034	.037	-.002	.022	.039	-.040	.011
v3	-.028	-.010		-.026	-.009	-.043	-.061	.071	.078	-.024	.040	-.002	-.019	.022
v4	.051	-.075	-.026		.112	-.043	.056	.006	-.042	.011	-.031	-.053	.038	-.025
v5	-.001	-.044	-.009	.112		-.010	.046	-.025	-.037	.060	-.044	-.022	.004	-.038
v6	-.024	.055	-.043	-.043	-.010		.108	-.012	.007	-.018	-.005	.004	.023	-.003
v7	.029	.021	-.061	.056	.046	.108		-.106	-.055	.031	-.070	-.034	.066	-.032
v8	.018	-.034	.071	.006	-.025	-.012	-.106		.021	-.016	.006	.031	-.017	.032
v9	-.053	.037	.078	-.042	-.037	.007	-.055	.021		-.015	.058	.028	-.048	.026
v10	-.001	-.002	-.024	.011	.060	-.018	.031	-.016	-.015		-.001	-.020	-.009	.001
v11	-.023	.022	.040	-.031	-.044	-.005	-.070	.006	.058	-.001		.097	-.037	-.012
v12	-.009	.039	-.002	-.053	-.022	.004	-.034	.031	.028	-.020	.097		-.044	-.010
v13	.026	-.040	-.019	.038	.004	.023	.066	-.017	-.048	-.009	-.037	-.044		.054
v14	-.018	.011	.022	-.025	-.038	-.003	-.032	.032	.026	.001	-.012	-.010	.054	

Extraction Method: Principal Axis Factoring.

b. Residuals are computed between observed and reproduced correlations. There are 19 (20.0%) nonredundant residuals with absolute values greater than 0.05.

FIGURE 9.8. Residual correlation matrix.

155

by sample sizes where very large sample sizes will produce statistical significance even with rather small loadings. In fact, each of the methods for determining lower bounds for adequate factor loadings is influenced by sample size. Thus, a potential solution would be for researchers to determine what percentage of variation in item response they hypothesize or theorize is sufficient for a factor to explain and take the square root. For example, if a researcher wishes for a factor to explain at least 25% of the variance in the responses to an item, then the lower bound for acceptable loadings should be the square root of 0.25, or 0.5. The initial factor loadings from the job satisfaction instrument are shown in Figure 9.9.

Factor Matrix[a]

	Factor	
	1	2
v1	.776	.282
v2	.587	.323
v3	.639	.434
v4	.761	.114
v5	.793	.088
v6	.668	.179
v7	.549	.128
v8	.746	.166
v9	.634	.337
v10	.762	-.334
v11	.739	-.387
v12	.761	-.397
v13	.691	-.360
v14	.776	-.358

Extraction Method: Principal Axis Factoring.[a]

a. 2 factors extracted. 5 iterations required.

FIGURE 9.9. Sample unrotated factor solution with two factors.

Clearly, these loadings violate the simple structure principle, but fortunately, we can adjust the loadings to better meet simple structure. This adjustment is called rotation and is the focus of the next section.

Rotation

To this point in the analysis, a researcher has conducted PAF depending on his or her purpose, has determined a number of factors to extract, and has a table of factor loadings. However, the factor loadings may not yet be easily interpreted. Anyone who has ever been to the theatre, concert, sporting event, or similar activity where one is seated in a large crowd probably knows that there is no guarantee of a clear view of the stage or playing field from one's seat. Yet, one most certainly knows that there are performers or athletes present despite the inability to actually see them. One might also end up moving from side to side in the hopes of finding a line of vision between the other patrons to catch a glimpse of the action. This analogy is similar to what rotation methods do with factor loadings. Rotation generally refers to the process of making a factor solution more interpretable without changing the actual underlying structure of the data (Mertler & Vannatta, 2005). In essence, the solution is adjusted to maximize simple structure (i.e., each item loading strongly onto only one factor). DeVellis (2012) described the purpose of rotation as increasing interpretability by identifying a set of items that have a relationship with only one and the same factor. Pedhazur and Schmelkin (1991) stated that Thurstone's concept of simple structure has had the "greatest impact on the development of various rotational approaches aimed at improving interpretability" (p. 612).

Factors and their associated items can be represented graphically where each factor is a dimension. Because most of us are better able to think in two-dimensional space, we will explain rotation methods using a two-factor solution. Think of each axis, x and y, as a factor using the job satisfaction dataset. Factor 1 (x-axis) represents the job characteristics factor, and Factor 2 (y-axis) represents the supervisory relationships factor. The unrotated factor loadings for each item can be used like coordinates to plot the item. For example, Item 1 in Figure 9.9 has a loading of 0.776 for Factor 1 and 0.282 on Factor 2. Thus, the coordinates for Item 1 are (0.776, 0.282).

Plotting all of the items in this manner produces the plot in Figure 9.10. As can be seen, interpreting the loadings with the placement of the axes would be very difficult. It might appear that both clusters of items load primarily on Factor 1, but this is not necessarily the case. By rotating the axes to produce the rotated factor loadings, interpretation becomes a

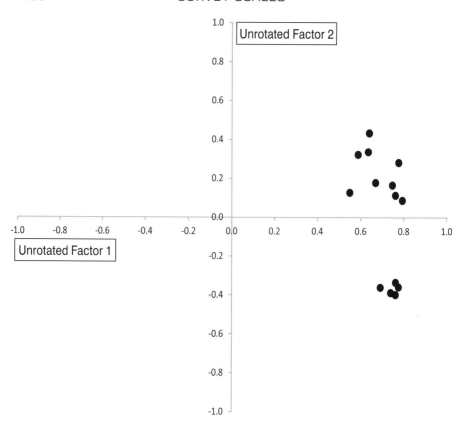

FIGURE 9.10. Factor loading plot for unrotated factor solution.

bit easier. With the rotation, the clusters of items are closer to their respective factor, which allows for easier interpretation.

When factors are hypothesized to be unrelated, the rotation method is referred to as orthogonal rotation, a term that comes from the Greek word meaning "right angled." In the rotation shown in Figure 9.10, the factors are not correlated to each other, which is why the axes are perpendicular. Orthogonal rotation is mathematically simpler and provides easier interpretation by researchers. Simply put, orthogonality is a restriction placed on the factor structure where the factors are kept independent of each other after rotation. Although several types of orthogonal rotation exist (e.g., quartimax, equimax, and varimax), the varimax type of rotation is by far the most commonly used. The rotation method is called varimax because it maximizes the variance of the standardized factor loadings summed across all factors. For technical details, see Comrey and Lee (1992), Gorsuch (1983), and Harman (1976).

Orthogonality is not a necessary condition for factor rotation, but solutions containing orthogonal factors will be easier to interpret. Rotation methods that allow factors themselves to be correlated are called oblique rotations. Unlike in orthogonal rotation, each axis in an oblique factor solution is essentially rotated separately around the origin but not necessarily to the same degree as the other axis or axes. In other words, the rotated axes may or may not be perpendicular. The relationship between factors obfuscates the interpretation of the factor loadings because items will load onto factors that are not necessarily fixed geometrically. That is, factor loadings are likely to be higher on all factors that are correlated because there is redundancy in the information contained by the factors (DeVellis, 2012). Given the difficulties of interpreting obliquely rotated solutions, it is not as frequently applied as are the orthogonal rotation methods. Yet, the decision regarding which rotation technique to employ should ultimately depend on the researcher's hypothesis and/or theory about the nature of the factors.

A reality is that factors are likely to be at least minimally correlated with each other regardless of theory or previous research. Therefore, competing strategies for addressing factor correlation have been proposed. Pedhazur and Schmelkin (1991) suggested researchers employ both orthogonal and oblique rotations in order to determine how strongly the factors are correlated. Stevens (2009) very conservatively stated that all factors are likely to be correlated to some degree, and it then is up to the researcher to identify the most appropriate oblique solution. If the correlation between factors is fairly small, then the researcher has provided evidence in favor of interpreting the orthogonal solution. Otherwise, the obliquely rotated solution should be considered. The primary oblique rotation techniques are promax and direct oblimin. As a reminder, both methods of rotation should be employed in a manner consistent with one's conceptual framework.

The rotated factor loadings using an oblique rotation method (i.e., promax) are shown in Figure 9.11, and the correlation between the factors is shown in Figure 9.12. The oblique structure seems to better produce simple structure, and the correlation between factors is 0.66, which is fairly strong. Based on all the information presented here, we selected the oblique rotated factor solution with two factors. The factor loading plot based on the rotated solution is shown in Figure 9.13. We should note that the axes in Figure 9.13 appear perpendicular because this is how plots are customarily presented; however, because of the correlation between the factors shown in Figure 9.13, the axes are actually *not* perpendicular. The concept of how the axes were rotated is shown in Figure 9.14.

Pattern Matrix[a]

	Factor	
	1	2
v1	.786	.058
v2	.727	-.090
v3	.891	-.200
v4	.574	.257
v5	.561	.306
v6	.599	.129
v7	.470	.129
v8	.629	.185
v9	.771	-.083
v10	.034	.809
v11	-.044	.862
v12	-.043	.887
v13	-.039	.804
v14	.013	.846

Extraction Method: Principal Axis Factoring.

Rotation Method: Promax with Kaiser Normalization.[a]

a. Rotation converged in 3 iterations.

FIGURE 9.11. Rotated factor solution with two factors.

Factor Correlation Matrix

Factor	1	2
1	1.000	.664
2	.664	1.000

Extraction Method: Principal Axis
Factoring.

Rotation Method: Promax with
Kaiser Normalization.

FIGURE 9.12. Factor correlation matrix from oblique rotation.

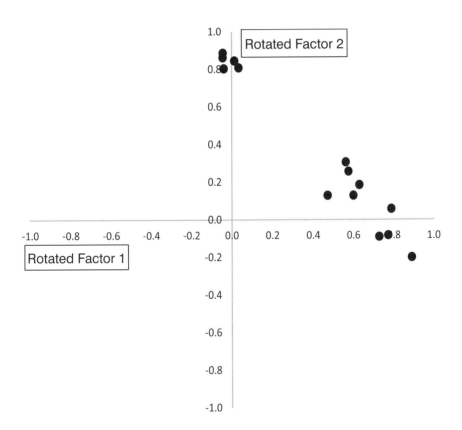

FIGURE 9.13. Factor loading plot for rotated factor solution.

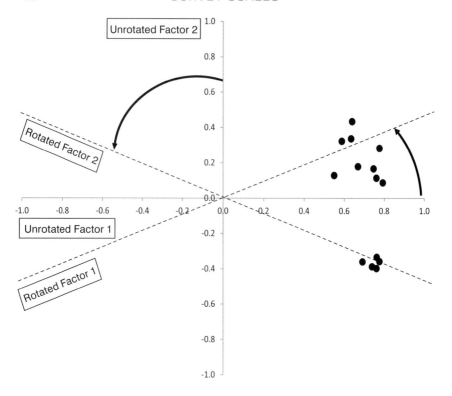

FIGURE 9.14. Conceptual representation of rotation with dashed lines representing the rotated axes.

How to Interpret Factor Solutions

At this point in the factor analysis, the major mathematical components of the procedure have been conducted, but the factors remain uninterpreted. Next, the researcher interprets the substantive meaning of the solution by examining the content of the items that load onto each factor. Based on the content of the items, the research would "name" the factor. Based on the obliquely rotated factor solution presented in Figure 9.11, Items 1 through 9 load most strongly onto the first factor and Items 10 through 14 load most strongly onto the second factor. Suppose those items were:

1. How satisfied are you with the overall working conditions here?
2. How satisfied are you with your work schedule?
3. How satisfied are you with the amount of responsibility you have?
4. How satisfied are you with the way this agency is managed?

5. How satisfied are you with the attention paid to suggestions you make?

6. How satisfied are you with your job security?

7. How satisfied are you with your job benefits?

8. How satisfied are you with how clearly your job responsibilities are defined?

9. Overall, how satisfied are you with your job as a direct service worker?

10. My supervisor is open to new and different ideas, such as a better way of dealing with care.

11. My supervisor is available to answer questions or advice when I need help with my clients.

12. My supervisor listens to me when I am worried about a client's care.

13. My supervisor tells me when I am doing a good job.

14. My supervisor is responsive with problems that affect my job.

Based on the content of these items, it seems that Items 1 through 9 are each related to some element of job satisfaction, and Items 10 through 14 are each related to some element of one's relationship with her or his supervisor. Therefore, one might reasonably name Factor 1 "job satisfaction" and Factor 2 "supervisory relationships."

Calculating Factor Scores

After the factors are named, researchers compute a score to represent how much of the construct is being represented in a person's responses. There are multiple methods for computing factor scores, and we will show how to get the factor scores using the factor solution shown in Figure 9.11. Perhaps the most common method is simply to sum the responses to items on each factor, which provides the factor sum score. Again as shown in Figure 9.11, Items 1 through 9 load onto Factor 1, and Items 10 through 14 load onto Factor 2. Suppose on Items 1 through 9, a respondent's coded responses were 4, 4, 3, 4, 3, 4, 4, 4, and 2, respectively. The same respondent's coded responses for Items 10 through 14 were 3, 3, 3, 4, and 3, respectively. Using the factor sum score method, the respondent would have a score of 32 (4 + 4+ 3 + 4 + 3 + 4 + 4 + 4 + 2 = 32) for Factor 1 and 16 (3 + 3 + 3 + 4 + 3 = 16) for Factor 2. This method is easy to conduct and interpret, and the sum score preserves variation in the data. The major disadvantages are that this treats ordinal-level data as if they were interval or ratio level, and each item is given equal weighting even though items may have different loadings.

A second method requires that a researcher rescale the item responses to have a specified mean and standard deviation before summing the rescaled item responses. Suppose a survey analyst wanted to standardize the items to have a mean of 0 and standard deviation of 1.0. She would rescale the items before summing them. Using the same items from the examples above, suppose the mean response for Item 1 is 4.5 and the standard deviation for Item 1 is 0.9. The respondent used in the example above would have a standardized score of

$$z = \frac{(4 - 4.5)}{0.9} = -0.56$$

The negative sign indicates that the respondent's score is below the overall item mean for item 1. This type of rescaling would be repeated for each of the 14 items using each item's mean and standard deviation. Finally, the sum scores would be computed for each factor like the previous example, except the standardized scores would be used instead of the actual coded responses. This method may be attractive when the variability in the item responses differs greatly, but this method also assigns equal weight to the items.

A third method requires the researcher to (1) rescale each item response as described above, (2) multiply the rescaled item response by the item loading, and (3) sum the products for all items loading onto each factor. We computed the standardized score for Item 1 above as 0.56, and the primary factor loading for Item 1 in Figure 9.12 is 0.786. To get the weighted score for Item 1 for the respondent, simply multiply the standardized score by the factor loading to get −0.440 (−0.56 × 0.786 = −0.440). Once again, this would be repeated for each of the 14 items. The weighted factor score for Factor 1 would be obtained by adding up the weighted scores of Items 1 through 9, and the weighted factor score for Factor 2 would be obtained by adding up the weighted scores of Items 10 through 14. This method recognizes the strength of the items, but as a result, it may be more heavily impacted by modeling decisions made by the researcher (e.g., rotation, variable selection). For many intents and purposes, computing simple sum scores for each factor may be sufficient. DiStefano, Zhu, and Mîndrilă (2009) provide an excellent discussion of each of the factor scoring methods.

Sample Size

In planning to complete a factor analysis to investigate the structure of your survey scale, you might ask how many survey respondents need to complete the scale to have enough data to conduct the analysis. Given the mathematical complexity of factor analysis and the amount of information needed to yield a reliable, or stable, factor-analytic solution, the astute reader would intuit the requirement of a large dataset. Many guidelines for minimum adequate sample size have been proposed for conducting factor analysis; these guidelines commonly involve maintaining a certain number of responses per item, obtaining a minimum sample size regardless of the number of items, or some combination of both. Crocker and Algina (2006), for example, noted a commonly regarded recommendation of the larger of 10 survey respondents per item and 100 total respondents. Tabachnick and Fidell (2013) recommended at least 300 survey respondents but preferably 500 to 1,000. They make no reference to the respondent-to-item ratio. Clearly, there is not one universally accepted guideline for minimum adequate sample size, but larger sample sizes are generally viewed as more desirable. It is critical to note that these recommendations will not apply to all studies. Other factors beyond the scope of this chapter may need to be considered. Interested readers should see MacCallum, Widaman, Zhang, and Hong (1999) and MacCallum, Widaman, Preacher, and Hong (2001) for an excellent discussion of these considerations.

Steps after EFA

After a factor solution is selected and interpreted, a powerful piece of validity evidence is to conduct confirmatory factor analysis (CFA) using an independent sample. If the factorial structure holds across multiple samples, then the researcher has evidence that the solution selected in the exploratory study was not an artifact of that particular sample.

As opposed to EFA, the researcher submits a specific solution to CFA and evaluates the adequacy of model fit through a series of statistical criteria and parameter estimates. Several software packages have CFA capabilities, of which AMOS, EQS, LISREL, Mplus, R, SAS, and Stata seem to be the most popular. The details of CFA are beyond our coverage in this book; interested readers should see Brown (2015) and Kline (2015) for a masterful coverage of CFA and other latent variable topics.

How to Obtain an EFA Model

Let's use SPSS to review the steps in conducting a factor analysis. With a dataset open in SPSS, click the Analyze menu, then Dimension Reduction, then Factor. . . . This will open the Factor Analysis dialogue box. Next, move each of the variables you wish to factor-analyze into the "Variables" box (see Figure 9.15). To obtain the reproduced and residual correlation matrices, you must open the "Descriptives . . ." options, select "Reproduced"

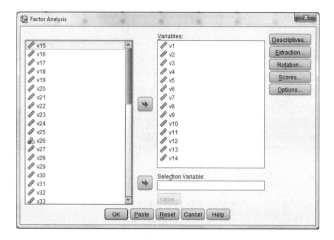

FIGURE 9.15. Screen shot of the Factor Analysis dialogue box.

(see Figure 9.16), and click "Continue" to close the Descriptives options. Principal axis factoring is not the default extraction method in SPSS, so you must next open the "Extraction . . ." options. In the Extraction options, select "Principal axis factoring" from the Method drop-down menu and also make sure the "Scree plot" option is checked (see Figure 9.17). Click "Continue" to close the Extraction options. Open the "Rotation . . ." options next. Select either the "Promax" or "Direct Oblimin" option to allow the factors to be correlated. If you discover after running the factor analysis that your factors are not correlated or very weakly correlated, you will simply rerun the factor analysis but select "Varimax" instead. See

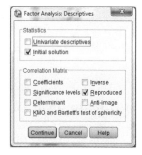

FIGURE 9.16. Screen shot of the Descriptives options in factor analysis. Reprinted courtesy of International Business Machines Corporation. Copyright © International Business Machines Corporation.

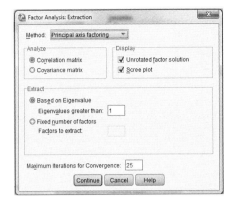

Figure 9.18 for a screenshot of Rotation options specifying the Promax rotation method. Click "Continue" to close the Rotation options. For most users with complete data, these are all of the options that need to be specified in order to run factor analysis. Click "OK" to run the factor analysis. If you wish/need to change any options, simply repeat these steps and make the necessary changes.

When choosing the Promax or Direct Oblimin rotation method, users are given the option to change Kappa or Delta, respectively. Kappa and Delta in this context are indices that control the level of correlation between factors one is willing to allow. The default values will likely be acceptable

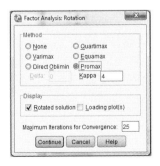

in most cases, but users should know both what the default values are and that they can be changed if necessary. The default number of iterations for convergence is 25. In certain instances, increasing the number of iterations may help users reach a solution, but it may also increase the computing time. In most cases, the default settings are likely acceptable.

In Chapter 10, we discuss methods for documentation of the scale development. Whether displaying the results of an analysis in something as simple as a frequency table or as complex as a factor loading plot, the results of the analyses must be presented in a manner that facilitates researchers' understanding of patterns in the data and communicates the findings to readers. We also examine the use of tables and figures in exploring the data and communicating results.

FURTHER READING

Comrey, A. L., & Lee, H. B. (1992). *A first course in factor analysis.* Hillsdale, NJ: Erlbaum.

> *Excellent but challenging introductory text on various factor-analytic components, including estimation algorithms, rotation methods, and design considerations.*

Gorsuch, R. L. (1983). *Factor analysis* (2nd ed.). Hillsdale, NJ: Erlbaum.

> *Classic introductory text on technical details of factor analysis. Excellent presentation of details and considerations for conducting factor analysis.*

Harman, H. H. (1976). *Modern factor analysis* (3rd ed.). Chicago: University of Chicago Press.

> *Another classic text on the technical details of factor analysis. Provides in-depth discussions of various approaches to estimation, rotation, and other details for conducting factor analysis.*

CHAPTER EXERCISES

1. A survey researcher has developed a survey scale that measures a construct composed of two dimensions. Review the eigenvalues, scree plot, and factor loadings below. Does the information support the researcher's conceptualization of a two-factor construct?

Total Variance Explained

Factor	Initial Eigenvalues Total	Initial Eigenvalues % of Variance	Extraction Sums of Squared Loadings Total	Extraction Sums of Squared Loadings Total	Extraction Sums of Squared Loadings % of Variance	Extraction Sums of Squared Loadings Cumulative %	Rotation Sums of Squared Loadings[a] Total
1	7.921	66.009	7.287	7.625	63.542	63.542	7.287
2	.996	8.302	6.438	.517	4.312	67.854	6.438
3	.526	4.387					
4	.449	3.743					
5	.350	2.914					
6	.313	2.606					
7	.287	2.392					
8	.280	2.330					
9	.253	2.106					
10	.235	1.955					
11	.207	1.722					
12	.184	1.534					

Extraction Method: Principal Axis Factoring.

a. When factors are correlated, sums of squared loadings cannot be added to obtain a total variance.

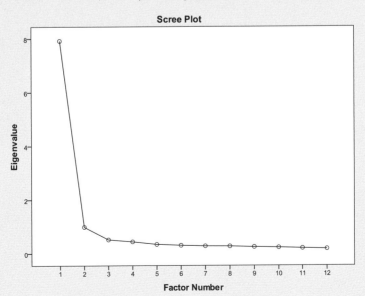

Scree Plot

Pattern Matrix[a]

	Factor	
	1	2
i1	.984	-.472
i2	.624	.280
i3	.613	.280
i4	.631	.271
i5	.561	.363
i6	.724	.146
i7	.712	.174
i8	.634	.266
i9	.659	.216
i10	.608	.265
i11	-.272	.974
i12	-.105	.787

Extraction Method: Principal Axis
Factoring.
Rotation Method: Promax with
Kaiser Normalization.[a]
a. Rotation converged in 3
iterations.

Factor Correlation Matrix

Factor	1	2
1	1.000	.802
2	.802	1.000

Extraction Method: Principal Axis
Factoring.
Rotation Method: Promax with
Kaiser Normalization.

2. Revisit the review of the Index of Teaching Stress (ITS) in Chapter 2.
What did the reviewer of the ITS report about the results of the factor
analysis of the instrument?

Documenting the Development of the Survey Scale

Many tables of data are badly presented. It is as if their producers
either did not know what the data were saying or were not letting on.
—Ehrenberg (1977, p. 277)

Introduction

Researchers often use tables and graphs to organize and display information for purposes of development, exploration, and communication (APA,
2010; Wainer, 1997). However, as Ehrenberg noted, the presentations
of the data have not always been optimal. Although you might consider
Ehrenberg's criticism a bit harsh, his characterization of the state of the
art in developing tables is supported by his colleagues. Over a century ago,
Arthur and Henry Farquhar (1891) wrote, "Getting information from a
table is like extracting sunlight from a cucumber" (p. 55). More recently,
Wainer (1992) wrote, "Tables, spoken of so disparagingly by the Farqu-
hars, remain, to a large extent, worthy of contempt" (p. 18).

Criticisms aside, if appropriately constructed, tables and graphs can
inform the survey scale developer's review of the survey data from a field
test and document the instrument construction. Technical reports provide
the potential user of a survey scale with information related to item quality and reliability and validity evidence (AERA et al., 2014). Also, recall
in Chapter 2 Nitko (n.d.) stated that in review sets of instruments, the
publisher should provide descriptions of the instrument content and a
rationale behind its selection; materials related to scoring, reporting, and

interpreting instrument results; the cost of the materials and scoring; and technical information (e.g., reliability and validity) about the instrument.

This type of information is not limited to technical reports; rather, documentation might serve as the description of the instrumentation in the Method section of a research article, a dissertation, or an evaluation report.

Preparation of the documentation for your scale requires consideration of the methods best suited for purposes of instrument development, data exploration, and communication of results. As we describe in Chapter 10, tables and graphs have the potential to contribute to the documentation process. We present guidelines in developing tables and graphs that will assist survey scale developers and researchers to explore patterns in the data; to examine item quality, validity, and reliability; and to communicate the survey results to readers.

Determining the Need for a Data Display

A first guideline in developing data displays is determining the need for a table or a graph. An important criterion in determining the need for a data display is whether it will help a survey developer to review the quality of the scale, a researcher to understand the survey data, or a reader to comprehend the survey findings (Evergreen, 2014).

Another guideline is to avoid using a table or graph when the information is limited (Few, 2004). For example, in Chapter 7, we discussed conducting statistical analyses by groups, such as males and females. In this instance, reporting the number of male and female survey participants would be best done in the text, and no table is required. If, however, you have the means for 35 items from a survey scale to organize and study patterns in the data, then a table or graph will be of benefit.

If a data display appears beneficial, then a next decision is whether a table or graph is appropriate. Tables can organize more data in less space than graphics. Table 10.1 contains field test data about teacher and preservice teacher performance on a web-based survey about ethics and assessment practices. The table provides (1) information about content areas (e.g., communication about grading), (2) a description of each content area, (3) examples of survey items, (4) the overall understanding of preservice and inservice teachers (i.e., Total), (5) preservice teacher understanding, and (6) teacher understanding.

However, sometimes a table cannot provide a visual that is as powerful as a graph. Figure 10.1 clearly shows the similarities of preservice and inservice teachers' performance within a content area. It also shows the differences of the preservice and inservice teachers' understanding across content areas. Both groups, for example, have a strong understanding of communication about grading (i.e., preservice teachers 89% correct, inservice

TABLE 10.1. Preservice and Inservice Teachers Percentage Correct Scores on Ethics and Classroom Assessment Items: An Example of Arranging Comparative Data by Columns

Content areas	Description	Example items	Total %	Preservice teachers %	Inservice teachers %
Communication about Grading	Providing information to students about the determination of grades	A middle school principal directs teachers to give students a written policy that explains how report card grades are calculated in their classes.	89	89	90
Multiple Assessment Opportunities	Using varied forms of assessments	A teacher assesses student knowledge by using many types of assessments: multiple-choice tests, essays, projects, portfolios.	87	87	87
Confidentiality	Protecting privacy of test results	To motivate students to perform better, a science teacher always announces that he is passing out scored tests to students in order of points earned, from the top score to the bottom score.	86	86	86
Standardized Test Administration	Implementing district and state testing procedures	While administering a standardized test, a teacher notices that a child has missed a problem that the student obviously knows. The teacher stands by the child's desk, taps her finger by the incorrect problem, shakes her head, and walks on to the next desk.	79	79	77
Bias	Maintaining fairness in assessment	A teacher allows a student with a learning disability in the language arts to use a tape-recorder when the student answers the essay questions on social studies tests.	64	66	60
Grading Practices	Assessing and scoring student learning	A teacher considers a student's growth in assigning grades.	51	51	52
Standardized Test Preparation	Preparing students for district and state testing	A teacher spends a class period to train his students in test-taking skills (e.g., not spending too much time on one problem, eliminating impossible answers, guessing).	37	34	46
Overall %			70	70	71

Note. Preservice teachers *n* = 77; inservice teachers *n*= 28.

173

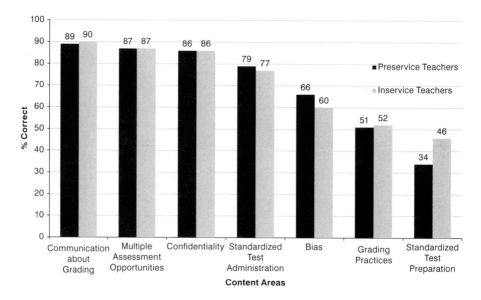

FIGURE 10.1. Inservice and preservice teachers' percentage correct on items related to the ethics of assessment practices in the classroom.

teachers 90% correct), and both groups need a better understanding of appropriate practices in preparing students for standardized testing (i.e., preservice teachers 34% correct, inservice teachers 46% correct). In the following sections, we provide guidelines for the development of tables and graphs.

Developing Tables

A table is a structure that displays numerical or textual information in columns and rows (APA, 2010; Few, 2004). The arrangement in rows and columns reveals patterns and exceptions. As seen in Table 10.2, a title accompanies the table and provides the reader with a concise explanation of the content of the table—in this instance, a comparison between the pass/fail status of students and their responses to items that gauge student engagement. Column headers and rows classify the data into variables for comparisons. In the example, the variables are pass/fail status and social engagement items from a survey scale. The data form the body of the table and consist of item means.

As discussed in Chapter 8, Table 10.2 provides validity evidence about criterion groups that are expected to differ with respect to the construct

TABLE 10.2. Means for Items on the Social Engagement Scale by Students Pass/Fail Status in Mathematics: An Example of the Structure of a Table

As a ninth-grade student I . . .	Fail	Pass	Total
care if I finish high school.	3.8	3.9	3.9
know my way around the school.	3.8	3.6	3.6
have many friends at school.	3.5	3.7	3.6
know what my teachers expect of me.	3.3	3.3	3.3
care what teachers think about me.	2.6	2.9	2.9
talk with adults (teachers, counselors, coaches) when I have problems.	2.5	2.7	2.7
care what other students think about me.	2.3	2.4	2.4
come to school only because my friends are here.	2.0	2.0	2.0
often get sent to an administrator for misbehaving.[a]	1.7	1.4	1.4
Overall mean	2.8	2.9	2.9

Note. Students failing mathematics $n = 31$; students passing mathematics $n = 147$. Item response scale: 1 = Strongly disagree, 2 = Agree, 3 = Agree, and 4 = Strongly agree. Adapted from Johnson, Davis, Fisher, Johnson, and Somerindyke (2000). Copyright © 2000 Richland School District Two, Columbia, South Carolina. Adapted by permission.
[a]Item uses negative wording and a low mean indicates positive student behavior.

of student engagement. If students are earning a pass in their mathematics class, then we might posit that they will have higher means on student engagement items than students who are failing their mathematics class. For five of the nine items, the mean is slightly higher for the students who are passing. Thus, the table allowed us to quickly surmise that the two criterion groups differed only slightly on the construct being measured. Considerations for developing a table include (1) the structure of tables and (2) the data to include in a table in order to convey the patterns contained in the survey responses.

Table Structure

To develop a table that supports survey development, data exploration, and communication of results, one must first consider its structure. Table 10.3 lists guidelines that will assist you in developing the appropriate structure of a table.

TABLE 10.3. Guidelines for Developing the Structure of a Table

- Determine the best way to organize the table.
- Order the table elements so the most important pattern is shown first and allows use of columns for comparisons.
- Place columns to be compared next to one another.
- Use spaces in tables to separate information clusters.
- Include all information required to comprehend a table within the display.
- Format comparable tables to be consistent in presentation.

Organization of the Table

A first consideration is determining the organization of a table that will convey the information in the data. For example, in Table 10.2, one option is to report the information using only the Total column; however, such a table would omit critical information needed to compare the engagement of students who are failing mathematics and students who are passing.

Should this information be further disaggregated by including student gender to determine if item means are lower for males or females? The answer depends on the purpose of your research. If your research is to study whether the construct of engagement is expressed differently for males and females, then adding columns with item means for males and females might reveal additional patterns in the data.

Emphasis on the Most Important Pattern

Related to organization of the table is ordering the columns so that the most important pattern is shown first (Ehrenberg, 1977). Return to Table 10.2 and compare the Fail column and Pass column. As we noted, the means for approximately half of the items are slightly higher for the Pass group as compared to the Fail group. Such a pattern is evident only if the table is organized to emphasize the most important pattern, in this instance the important pattern being the association between lower item means on engagement and failing mathematics. Thus, the first column is Fail and has means ordered high to low.

Placement of the Columns

Also contributing to the organization of the table is placing the columns to be compared next to one another (APA, 2010). Columns specify the variables to be compared. Of interest in Table 10.2 is whether the students who are failing respond differently than students who are passing. Placement of the Fail/Pass columns adjacent to one another facilitates this comparison.

Use of Space

Further aiding organization of a table is the use of spaces to separate information clusters (APA, 2010; Ehrenberg, 1977; Wainer, 1992, 1997). The intent is to use spacing to guide the eye to make patterns evident. In Table 10.2, a space at the bottom of the table serves to separate the overall mean for the scale from the individual item means. This space allows the reader to determine which items, as compared to the overall mean, are relatively high, such as "care if I finish high school," or relatively low, such as "often get sent to an administrator for misbehaving."

Information to Include in a Table

In preparing a table, include all information required within the display that is necessary for a reader to comprehend the table (APA, 2010). The table should include a title that informs the reader about the focus of the table. Columns should all have headings (i.e., labels). Standard abbreviations and symbols for nontechnical terms and symbols (e.g., *M*, *SD*, %) may be used in table headings without explanation (APA, 2010). However, abbreviations that are unfamiliar to most readers should be avoided.

In the case of unfamiliar information that is critical, another option is to provide this information in the table notes (see Table 10.2). Use of table notes allows you to provide information relevant to the table as a whole (i.e., a general note); to focus on a specific column, row, or cell (i.e., a specific note); and to specify *p*-values (i.e., a probability note). The table note in Table 10.2 specifies the number of students who failed mathematics and the number who passed mathematics. Both the statement about the number of students failing/passing and the information about the response scale are general notes, whereas the information about the negatively worded item is a specific note and is identified by a superscript, lowercase letter.

Consistent Format of Comparable Tables

To facilitate comparisons across tables, format comparable tables to be consistent in presentation (APA, 2010). Thus, titles should be comparable, the structure of the rows and columns should be similar, and you should use the same headers (i.e., not synonyms). In this manner, the organization of the initial table can inform the development of subsequent tables. A word of caution is warranted: On occasion, to take advantage of the energy expended in developing an initial table, a researcher will force data into the table structure, even though the table will not display the intended patterns. So, consider the concurrence between the structure of a newly developed table and the patterns in the data that subsequent tables should display.

Table Data

Developing a useful table requires effective organization of the data. Guidelines for organization of the data are presented in Table 10.4.

Presentation of Data in Columns

If a table is to be used to make comparisons, then the data to be compared should be arranged into a column format because, as stated by Ehrenberg (1977), "Figures are easier to follow reading down a column than across a row, especially for a larger number of items" (p. 282). For example, returning to Table 10.1, if a researcher is investigating educators' understanding of ethical classroom assessment practices, then the percentage correct for *all* educators could be listed in the first column. This allows the survey developer to read down the first column to ascertain the difficulty (i.e., percentage correct) of the content areas and determine if the survey scale needs to add more demanding (i.e., difficult) items, or additional easier items, in order to increase the overall variability of the survey scale. Communication about Grading, for example, is a content area that needs additional challenging items.

In contrast, the data are formatted as a row in the partial display of Table 10.5. To compare educator understanding of the content categories, the eye must travel across the full page to read the data in the row, whereas the same information in a column is more compact and allows the reader to look at the differences between categories (e.g., the difference between

---

TABLE 10.4. Guidelines for the Organization of the Data in a Table

- Present data in columns to facilitate comparisons.
- Order the statistics from high to low, rather than by alphabetical order or the position of items in the survey scale.
- Include overall column and row statistics (e.g., item mean, totals) to allow comparisons.
- Round decimals to two place values (e.g., correlations).
- Report actual values for negatively worded items (i.e., do not report recoded values).

TABLE 10.5. Preservice and Inservice Teachers Percentage Correct Scores on Ethics and Classroom Assessment Items: An Example of Arranging Data by Row and the Difficulty of Comparison

Category	Communication about grading	Multiple assessment opportunities	Confidentiality	Standardized test administration	Bias	Grading practices	Standardized test preparation	Overall
Total % correct	89	87	86	79	64	51	37	70
Preservice teachers (N = 77)	89	87	86	79	66	51	34	70
Inservice teachers (N = 28)	90	87	86	77	60	52	46	71

Communication about Grading [89%] and Standardized Test Preparation [37%] being 52%).

The Order of Statistics

Rather than arranging data following the position of items in the survey scale, or arranging alphabetically by items, order the statistics so that the reader will see the critical patterns in the data. For example, in data exploration, a researcher might order the statistics from high to low to allow comparison between items (Ehrenberg, 1977; Wainer, 1992). Thus, for Table 10.2, you can see that students who failed mathematics indicated that they "know what my teachers expect of me" ($\bar{X} = 3.3$) but less often indicated they "care what teachers think about me" ($\bar{X} = 2.6$). If Table 10.1 had been arranged alphabetically, the area of Bias would be listed first and make it a little more difficult to detect the content area in which respondents demonstrate the most understanding, that is, Communication about Grading. Another way to arrange data is from past to present, as one might use to illustrate changes over time.

Column and Row Overall Statistics

Including overall column and row totals (or means) allows comparisons of a statistic, such as an item mean, with the statistics associated with other survey scale items (Ehrenberg, 1977; Wainer, 1992, 1997). In Table 10.2 the column totals of 2.8 for students failing mathematics and 2.9 for students passing mathematics show that overall the responses on the social engagement items were similar for both groups. In addition to item means, one might include medians and row or column totals.

Rounding to Two Place Values

Two issues should be considered in rounding the statistics in tables. First, when a statistical package is used to calculate the statistics for a scale, the output might calculate the statistics to four decimal points or more. However, it is doubtful that the data reflect this level of precision. The APA (2010) noted that fewer decimal digits are easier to comprehend than more and recommended rounding to two decimals (p. 113). In the item means for Table 10.2, we rounded to one decimal, making comparisons easier. Notice, for example, student response to the item "As a ninth-grade student I talk with adults (teachers, counselors, coaches) when I have problems." Carried to two decimal places, the item means are 2.52 (failing) and 2.69 (passing). Using the means with two decimals, we see that the difference is 0.17. If the means are rounded to one decimal, 2.5 and 2.7, a quick calculation shows the difference to be 0.2. Thus, rounding facilitates comparison.

Second, you should consider whether other numerical values should be rounded to two significant digits (Ehrenberg, 1977; Wainer, 1992, 1997). This recommendation is based on our inability to remember, understand, and mentally manipulate more than two digits. Wainer (1997) provided an example in which a school budget is reported as $27,329,681. He asked: "Who can comprehend or remember that? If we remember anything it is almost surely the translation 'This year's school budget is about 27 million dollars'" (p. 5). In addition, Wainer wrote that rounding unclutters a table and makes patterns more apparent.

However, Wainer (1997) provided another example that raises a caution. He presented a table that reported trends in population. The table showed the populations of Detroit and Los Angeles in 1920 as being 950,000 and 500,000, respectively. Wainer argued that the information would be more interpretable if the populations were rounded to two significant place values. Thus, when the units were labeled as being in the millions, the population information became 1.0 and 0.5, respectively. However, the reporting of 500,000 as 0.5 million raises questions about whether 0.5 million is readily understood by the reader to be 500,000. Our recommendation is consistent with that of Ehrenberg (1977): to round for presentation but not for calculations. But we add, round only to the extent that it enhances the reader's comprehension of the meaning of the data.

Reporting Statistics for Negatively Worded Items

On occasion, survey scale developers include negatively worded items in a scale. In Table 10.2, an example of a negatively worded item is "As a ninth-grade student I often get sent to an administrator for misbehaving." In Chapter 8 we discussed the need to reverse score the item prior to using it in an item analysis, adding it to a total score, or calculating internal consistency. The main precept behind using reverse scoring is the idea that as a total score increases, then the construct underlying the total score should increase. So, for a negatively worded item we want the total score to increase if the student *disagrees* with the statement. However, in reporting the item mean or frequencies, we recommend reporting the actual item values, not the recoded values. This is necessary because the reverse-scored item will confuse the reader. To continue our example, an overall item mean of 3 or 4 on a 4-point scale for being sent to an administrator for misbehaving would mislead the readers into thinking the school has a behavior problem.

Developing Graphs

A graph provides summary information through the use of bars or lines that display numerical information typically within an *x*- and *y*-axis. As with tables, the arrangement of a graph can reveal patterns in the data (Few, 2004). As seen in Figure 10.1, a caption accompanies the graph and provides the reader with a brief explanation about the figure—in this instance, a comparison of preservice and inservice teacher's percentage correct scores on a survey scale on ethics and classroom assessment practices.

Structure of a Graph

To develop a graph that supports exploration and communication, one must first consider its structure. The guidelines in Table 10.6 will assist you in considering the structure of a graph.

Choice of a Bar Graph or a Line Graph

The first guideline in Table 10.6 requires you to consider whether a bar graph or a line graph will best serve to explore the data or to convey the findings of a study. Bar graphs are useful for comparing groups. In Figure 10.1, the bar graphs allow comparison of two groups: preservice and inservice teachers. Particularly striking is the bar graphs' demonstration that preservice and inservice teachers had similar levels of understanding about ethics and classroom assessment practices. However, the graph also informed us that the preservice and inservice teachers' performance differed across content areas.

As shown in Figure 10.2, a line graph could be used instead of the bar graph. However, notice that the two lines (i.e., preservice and inservice teachers) overlap and that the similarities are not as visually striking in the

TABLE 10.6. Guidelines for Developing the Structure of a Graph
• Determine whether a bar graph or a line graph is needed.
• Label your x-axis and y-axis.
• Decide on the vertical and horizontal values of the scale axes.
• Determine the need for gridlines.
• Develop legends that describe the lines or bars in the graph.
• Place legends close to the elements they describe.
• Limit the number of bars and lines.
• Limit shading and keep it distinct.
• Avoid pie graphs, stacked bar graphs, and 3-D graphs.

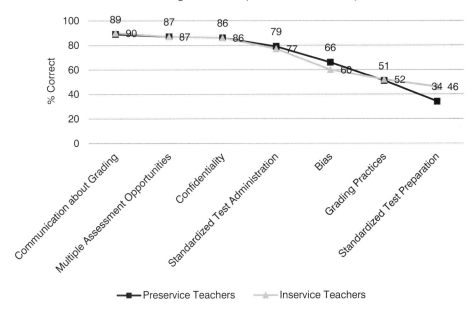

FIGURE 10.2. Inservice and preservice teachers' percentage correct on items related to the ethics and classroom assessment: Example of a line graph.

line graph as they are in the bar graph. A strength of line graphs is their use in depicting changes over time (Evergreen, 2014).

x-Axis and *y*-Axis Labels

As with tables, one goal in developing a graph is for the display to contain all the information required for the reader to understand the patterns depicted in the figure. Contributing to a reader's understanding is the use of labels to define the *x*- and *y*-axes (Fink, 2002). In Figure 10.1, the label for the *x*-axis is Content Areas, and for the *y*-axis it is % Correct. Taken together, the labels inform the reader that the graph provides information about the relationship between (1) content areas in ethics and classroom assessment (e.g., Communication about Grading, Multiple Assessment Opportunities) and (2) the percentage correct.

Vertical and Horizontal Values for the Scale Axes

Typically, the *y*-axis of a graph should begin at zero to avoid biasing the reader's perception (Evergreen, 2014; Few, 2004; Fink, 2002). Contrast Figure 10.3 with Figure 10.1. With the *y*-axis starting at 50% correct, the

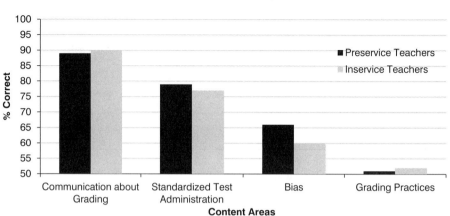

184

FIGURE 10.3. Inservice and preservice teachers' percentage correct on items related to the ethics and assessment practices: Example of distortion by truncation of the y-axis.

graph exaggerates the differences between inservice and preservice teachers in the area of Bias.

Need for Gridlines

Gridlines tend to clutter the graph (Evergreen, 2014). However, the use of light gray gridlines provides a link between the value on the vertical axis and the category on the horizontal axis. In Figure 10.4, the gridlines are light gray. A solid line is use to indicate performance level on a goal. In some evaluations, staff will set a goal for the agreement level of participants on Likert-style items. The black line indicates to the reader that the program set a goal of 80% agreement with items in a survey scale. At a glance, the reader sees that the goal was met for two items and not met on three items.

Legends

Legends also contribute to the readers' understanding of a graph. In Figure 10.1, we saw a traditional legend embedded in the graph. Consistent with the APA (2010) recommendation that labels be close to the elements they are describing, in Figure 10.5 the legend is part of the graphic (Evergreen, 2014). Notice that the preservice teacher and inservice teacher labels from the legend are now embedded in the black and gray bars, respectively. Together, the axis labels and the legend labels inform the reader about the relationship between the preservice teacher's and inservice teacher's understanding of the content areas in classroom assessment and ethics.

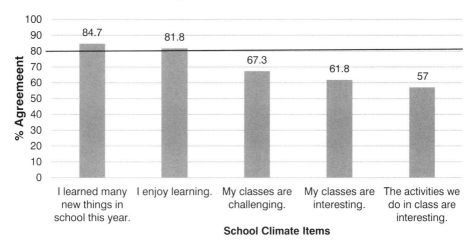

FIGURE 10.4. Percentage of student agreement (i.e., "Agree" and "Strongly agree") on items related to school climate: Use of a referent line.

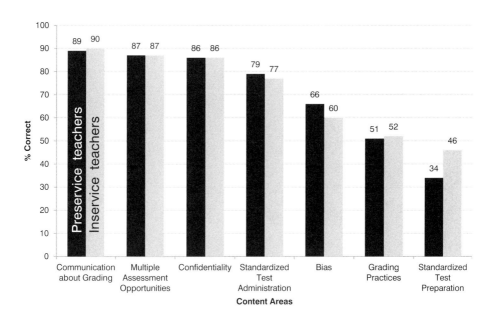

FIGURE 10.5. Inservice and preservice teachers' percentage correct on items related to the ethics of assessment practices in the classroom: Example of the labels for a legend being embedded in the bars of a graph.

Number of Bars and Lines

Fink (2002) recommended limiting the lines or bars in graphs to 4 or 5. Exceeding this number begins to clutter the graph and might interfere with the recognition of any patterns in the data. The bar graphs in Figure 10.5 make the data display busy but still allow the reader to see the pattern. Notice that in Figure 10.2 the overlap of the two lines makes the data values difficult to read.

Shading

Use of fill patterns for bar graphs or line styles for line graphs makes the interpretation of the information more difficult for the reader (Few, 2004). Vivid lines in the fill pattern create a visual vibration, a "jumpiness," for the reader, whereas breaks in the overlapping lines of a graph make it difficult to follow their flow. A remedy is to select an emphasis color, such as black, and to use a grayscale palate (Evergreen, 2014; Few, 2004). The palate should be used throughout the report.

According to Evergreen (2014), the background of the graph should be white. The white background allows you to use other shadings to make bars and lines in graphs distinct from one another. In addition, if gridlines are to be used in a graph, a white background allows you to use light gray gridlines to prevent the graph from becoming too cluttered. Figure 10.1 uses a white background, light gray gridlines, and black and gray bars to maintain a sharp image.

Graphs to Avoid

Graphs to avoid include pie graphs (Few, 2004), stacked bar graphs, and 3-D graphs (Evergreen, 2014; Few, 2004). Evergreen recommended avoiding pie charts because this type of graph depends on the readers' comprehension of area and readers do not easily interpret the area of a circle. Also, Wainer (2010) noted that readers' comparisons of segments in a pie are inaccurate.

Graphs presented in 3-D are difficult for the reader to comprehend, slowing down interpretation and decreasing accurate understanding (Evergreen, 2014). Clarity in interpretation is not achieved when interpreting a 3-D graph; for instance, the reader does not know whether to read from the front or the back of the bar (Evergreen, 2014).

We also recommend avoiding stacked bar graphs owing to the difficulty of understanding the relationship between the segments of the bar and the percentages that each segment represents. In Figure 10.6, although we collapsed the "Agree" and "Strongly agree" categories, and then arranged the bars from highest percentage to lowest percentage for those two categories,

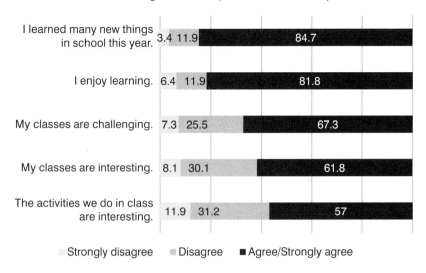

Strongly disagree   Disagree   Agree/Strongly agree

FIGURE 10.6. Percentage of student agreement on items related to school climate: Example of the use of a stacked bar graph.

the information is difficult to interpret. Contrast the demands in the interpretation of Figure 10.4 and Figure 10.6. A stacked bar graph might be appropriate if it is important to know the percentage breakdown for each response category (e.g., 8.1% "Strongly disagree," 30.1% "Disagree," 52.8% "Agree," and 9% "Strongly agree" for "My classes are interesting.").

Organization of Data in a Graph

Developing a useful graph requires effective organization of the data. Table 10.7 offers guidelines for organizing the data.

Ordering Bars and Lines to Highlight Important Patterns

One method to highlight patterns with bar and line graphs is to order bars from longest to shortest and lines from the highest point to the lowest point

TABLE 10.7. Guidelines for Organizing Data in a Graph
• Order the bars and lines to highlight the most important pattern.
• Place statistics at the end of the bars or adjacent to the data points in the lines.

(Evergreen, 2014). The bar graph in Figure 10.1 and the line graph in Figure 10.2 display the statistics from highest value to lowest value.

Location of Statistics

As shown in Figure 10.1, when possible, place statistics at the end of a bar in a bar graph (Evergreen, 2014). In the case of a line graph, place the statistics at each data point in the plot. This mode of formatting is consistent with the APA (2010) recommendation that labels be close to the elements they are describing.

Narrative about Table or Graph

Now that you have developed the tables and graphs to inform your analysis of the data or to communicate your findings to other researchers or to stakeholders in a program evaluation, a next step is to write text that describes and explains for the reader the patterns depicted in the tables and graphs (APA, 2010; Ehrenberg, 1977). Every table and figure must be accompanied by text that highlights the information to which the reader should attend (APA, 2010). Table 10.8 lists examples of types of text

TABLE 10.8. Types of Narrative That Describes and Explains Tables and Graphs

Function of text	Description
Introduction	Sets the stage for the report and provides information important for understanding of a table or graph.
Explanation	Provides information right at the point it is needed to clarify elements of a table or graph.
Reinforcement	Expresses information in more than one way, such as text and a table or graphic.
Highlighting	Emphasizes or calls attention to particular information by referencing with words.
Sequencing	Directs readers to navigate material in a particular order, such as read a conceptual framework in a particular way.
Recommendation	Suggest action based on report findings.
Inquiring	Raise questions and suggest further exploration and speculation based on the information from tables and graphs.

Note. Based on Few (2004, pp. 125–127).

typically associated with tables and graphs (Few, 2004). The information to be conveyed to the reader will determine the function of the text. For example, the purpose of the text accompanying a table might be to provide an explanation to clarify elements of the table. In contrast, the narrative might reinforce specific information in the table.

Concluding Thoughts

We opened *Survey Scales* with a quote from Chow (2010): "To conduct research is to collect, analyze, and interpret data systematically so as to answer specific questions about a phenomenon of interest" (p. 1260). Chow's statement illustrates the role of instrumentation and the data from that instrument in the conduct of research and evaluation. The guidance offered in *Survey Scales* will contribute to the development of a survey scale that will provide data to support you in drawing valid interpretations about your research focus. For example, adherence to the guidelines for writing items and developing response categories will contribute to the clarity of the items for the survey respondents. Their responses, in turn, will provide you with data that accurately reflect respondents' attitudes, knowledge, and behaviors. The chapter on descriptive statistics, Chapter 7, allows us to make informed choices about the appropriate type of statistical analyses to use in examining the quality of scales and items in those scales. All is for naught, though, if in the presentation of the data we lose our readers, so we examined methods for reporting to your audience (e.g., fellow survey developers and researchers) in a manner that conveys your research findings. Thus, the guidelines presented in *Survey Scales* provide a framework for the development of an instrument to assist in the collection, analysis, and interpretation of data in order to answer research questions about a phenomenon of interest.

FURTHER READING

Evergreen, S. (2014). *Presenting data effectively: Communicating your findings for maximum impact.* Thousand Oaks, CA: Sage.

   Presents guidelines in developing tables and graphs that inform the researchers and communicate research findings to the reader.

CHAPTER EXERCISES

1. Review the table below. How can the table be improved? In your answer, consider the utility of the table in making patterns more evident for a researcher or an evaluator and clearly communicating the findings to the reader. Also, consider the guidelines in the APA style manual.

Classroom Assessments Used to Monitor Student's Reading Progress	
70.20%	Anecdotal notes
60.30%	Core reading tests (supplied by publisher)
41.80%	Miscue analysis
52.60%	Vocabulary tests
67.60%	Spelling tests
97.90%	Writing samples
88.40%	Kidwatching/observation
65.00%	Running records
92.70%	Conferencing with students
65.80%	Teacher-made tests (e.g., multiple choice, short answer, matching)
65.30%	Student portfolios

2. Compare the table and bar graph below. Both are based on the same data. What does the figure communicate about trends more quickly than the table? How can each be improved?

Student Ratings on the Student–Teacher Interaction Scale by Pass and Fail for Mathematics						
Student–Teacher Interactions	Pass			Fail		
	N	Mean	SD	N	Mean	SD
My math teacher calls students by their names.	208	3.65	0.65	87	3.55	0.73
My math teacher has a sense of humor.	209	2.69	0.96	86	2.28	1.08
My math teacher tries to be helpful.	202	3.32	0.84	87	2.87	0.99

My math teacher cares about what students have to say.	206	2.99	0.90	86	2.53	0.94
My math teacher compliments student successes.	208	3.00	0.95	87	2.64	1.00
My math teacher puts students down for mistakes.	209	1.54	0.81	87	1.85	0.92

Adapted from Johnson, Davis, Fisher, Johnson, and Somerindyke (2000), Copyright © 2000 Richland School District Two, Columbia, South Carolina. Adapted by permission.

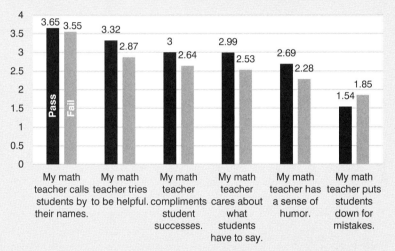

3. Review the types of text that Few (2004) indicated are used to describe tables and graphs. Which type(s) of narrative would you use to describe the table in the previous item about student–teacher interaction?

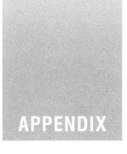

Analysis of Data

INFERENTIAL STATISTICS

By a small sample, we may judge the whole piece.
—MIGUEL DE CERVANTES

Introduction

In this Appendix, we describe the use of inferential statistics when analyzing data collected from survey scales. It provides guidelines for parametric (i.e., *t*-tests, analysis of variance) and nonparametric (i.e., Wilcoxon–Mann–Whitney, Kruskal–Wallis) procedures for analyzing differences between two or more groups. Confidence intervals and measures of **effect size** for these procedures also will be presented. In addition, readers will gain practice interpreting the results given the assumptions of each statistical test presented.

In Chapter 7, we discussed descriptive statistics as used to describe a particular set of data. Inferential statistics, in contrast, are used to make decisions or inferences about a broader collection of people, also known as a population. In statistics, a population refers to all subjects or members of a group who share one or more characteristics of interest. The primary goal of researchers in many cases is to learn something about a population or to make statements about some characteristic of a population. For example, a researcher comparing high school students in two districts might be interested in examining the students' average levels of perceived career readiness. Numerical values used to describe populations are called **parameters**. Thus, the mean level of perceived career readiness for the population of high school students would be considered a parameter because it describes all students.

Sampling

In reality, it is typically not feasible to survey and collect data from every student or member of a population. Technically, missing data from only a single student would prevent a population parameter from being calculated. Instead, researchers rely on samples, which are subsets of subjects or members who are derived from a population. Numerical values used to describe samples, such as those presented in Chapter 7, are called statistics and are considered estimates of population parameters.

The best sample is the one that is most representative of its parent population, but there are many methods available for sampling people from a population. Sampling methods that involve randomness are likely to result in more representative samples in the long run. Randomness should not be taken to mean that the sampling is haphazardly conducted or done without planning. Instead, random sampling implies that every member of a population has a random chance of being selected. As a result, any differences between the sample and population will be unsystematic, which is desired. In essence, random sampling helps minimize selection bias in the sample in the long run.

An example will help illustrate the importance of minimizing sampling bias. Suppose a researcher wanted to study the impact of a lateral entry teacher preparation program on students' views of teacher–student interaction. A sample is selected that includes students with teachers from lateral entry teacher preparation programs and students with teachers from traditional preparation programs. The students will complete a survey scale designed to measure various aspects of interaction between the teacher and students. Consider the implications on the study if somehow students who had more negative views of teacher–student interaction had a higher chance of being selected than students with positive perceptions. If this form of sampling bias occurred for students in the lateral entry teachers' classes, then chances are the analysis using the sample's data would falsely suggest that the lateral entry program is ineffective in fostering positive interaction between its teachers and their students. Such a scenario demonstrates the effect sampling bias has on inferences made based on a sample. Strategies can be put in place to ensure that samples are more representative of the population. Interested readers should see Cochran (1977) and Jaeger (1984) for a detailed discussion of various sampling methods and strategies.

When a sample is drawn from a population, the values of each variable (e.g., scores from a survey scale) from the members of the sample make up a distribution and are ordered from lowest to highest for continuous variables. Each sample's distribution can be described using the statistics presented in Chapter 7. That is, each distribution will have its own mean, standard deviation, and other characteristics. If a new sample containing the same number of subjects is drawn from a population, then the distribution for the second sample is likely to have similar characteristics as that of the first but is not likely to be *exactly* the same. Therefore, each sample's mean, standard deviation, and so on, will be slightly different than those estimates from other samples. If one repeatedly drew samples of the same size (i.e., same number of members), then the researcher would obtain a distribution of statistics. For example, if a researcher drew 100 random samples from a population, then she would have 100 means (i.e., one from each sample). Such a collection of statistics is referred to as a sampling distribution. A sampling distribution can be constructed for a mean, median, standard deviation, a correlation coefficient, difference between two means, or any number of other statistics.

Just as the distribution of the values of a variable taken from members of a sample has a mean and standard deviation, so does a sampling distribution. The mean of a sampling distribution is said to be equal to the population parameter. The standard deviation of the sampling distribution is referred to as the **standard error**. Standard error is essential in inferential statistical procedures. Recall from Chapter 7 that a standard deviation represented the typical distance of a value in a distribution from the sample mean. Conceptually, the interpretation of standard error is similar, given that it is the standard deviation of the sampling distribution. The standard error reflects how far each sample mean is away from the expected population mean, given the sample size.

Sample size is another important element in understanding standard errors. Larger samples are more likely to yield sample means that are closer to the expected population mean because it is less likely for a random sample to be composed of many people whose scores are far from the mean. In other words, repeatedly drawing very large random samples will likely produce a sampling distribution with less variability. Conversely, repeatedly drawing a sample of only two people is more likely to produce a sampling distribution with more variation. Thus, a collection of means based on small samples is likely to have larger differences overall than a collection of means taken from the larger samples.

This is easily seen by using the formula for standard error. The sample mean is the most commonly used statistic for making comparisons; so this example is based on the standard error of the mean. The standard error of the mean can be expressed as: $s_{\bar{x}} = s/\sqrt{n}$, where s is the standard deviation estimate from a sample and n is the sample size. For illustration purposes, suppose that the standard deviation of a sample of survey scores is equal to 10. The standard error of the mean based on a sample size of 100 is estimated to be 1 (i.e., $10/\sqrt{100} = 1$). The standard error estimate based on a sample size of 16 is 2.5 (i.e., $10/\sqrt{16} = 2.5$). Notice that even though both samples have a standard deviation of 10, the smaller sample of 16 is associated with more error (i.e., 2.5) and the larger sample of 100 with less error (i.e., 1.0).

Inferential Statistics

The principles presented above provide the basis for the use of inferential statistics via hypothesis or statistical significance testing. Inferential statistics incorporate sample statistics in conjunction with standard errors so that researchers may reach decisions about the population parameters in which they are ultimately interested. You might have noticed the frequent use of the term "likely" in the discussion on standard errors. The term "likely" is associated with the concept of "likelihood" or probability. Making decisions through hypothesis testing is based on the probability or likelihood of getting a particular sample statistic when the researcher holds certain conditions to be true. In the following sections, hypothesis testing will be presented along with several inferential statistical procedures that are frequently used when comparing groups of people, such as in program evaluation in education, health care, and related fields.

Hypothesis Testing

One method for making determinations about the population parameters based on the sample data collected is hypothesis testing. The importance of having a representative sample should be reinforced here. In hypothesis testing, the researcher conducts a statistical test that assists with determining the value of the population parameter of interest. The test about the population parameter is based on two mutually exclusive hypotheses: the **null hypothesis** and the **alternative hypothesis**. The difference between two groups' means (μ_D) is a common parameter of interest in hypothesis testing and will be used to illustrate the following definitions. Using the difference between two group means, we find that the null hypothesis which is denoted by H_0, would state that the two means are exactly the same, or the difference is equal to zero (H_0: $\mu_D = 0$). Still another way of stating the null hypothesis under the difference between the two group means scenario is that the two samples were drawn from the same population. If the two groups were drawn from the same population, then there will be no differences between their means. More generally, the null hypothesis states that there is no effect of an independent variable (e.g., treatment, intervention).

The alternative hypothesis, which is denoted as H_1, opposes the null hypothesis by specifying how the null hypothesis is false. For example, the alternative hypothesis when testing the equality of group means might state that a difference between the group means is not equal to zero. Note that this alternative hypothesis does not specify which group has a higher or lower mean. This is called a nondirectional alternative hypothesis. If the researcher had specified an alternative hypothesis that, say, Group 1 had a higher mean than Group 2, then it would be a directional hypothesis.

With the hypotheses specified, the researcher makes a decision based on the data about the probability that the sample was drawn from a population consistent with the null hypothesis. In hypothesis testing, it is the null hypothesis that is being tested because it is easier for the researcher to provide evidence against the null hypothesis than in favor of the alternative hypothesis.

The next step in hypothesis testing involves finding the probability of obtaining the sample observations (or observations more extreme) if the null hypothesis is true. This is where standard error plays a crucial role. Recall that the standard error is the typical amount of deviation between statistics in the sampling distribution. Under the current example, the parameter of interest is the mean difference between two groups. The researcher then takes the difference between the mean difference observed in the sample and the population parameter hypothesized under the null hypothesis (i.e., 0) and divides that difference by the standard error. Doing so returns a value, called a test statistic, that allows the researcher to determine the probability of observing a value of a test statistic, or one more extreme, assuming the null hypothesis is true. This probability is widely known as the p-value. If the p-value is very small, then the researcher might decide to reject the null hypothesis. Rejecting the null hypothesis is associated with statistical significance. If the p-value is relatively large, then the researcher might conclude that he or she does not have sufficient evidence to reject the null hypothesis. Note that a researcher is never completely sure that his or her decision is correct.

Rejecting the null hypothesis owing to a small p-value depends on a very important specification on the part of the researcher. That is, how small is small enough? The probability below which a p-value must fall in order to conclude that results are statistically significant is called the Type I error rate, which is commonly denoted as α. That is, what risk of making the incorrect decision is the researcher willing to accept in hypothesis testing? In social science research, the Type I error rate is commonly set at 5%, meaning that a researcher is only willing to assume a 5% chance of rejecting a true null hypothesis. If the researcher rejects a true hypothesis (i.e., concluding that there is a difference when there is in fact not a difference), then he has committed a Type I error.

Researchers can also make the opposite mistake. They can fail to reject a null hypothesis that should be rejected. In other words, a researcher may conclude that two groups' means are equivalent when they are not. Such an error is referred to as Type II error, and the Type II error rate is denoted with β. The probability of rejecting a false null hypothesis is referred to as statistical power, and power can be calculated by subtracting β from 1 (i.e., $1 - \beta$ = statistical power). Information regarding correct decisions and Type I and II errors in hypothesis testing are summarized in Table A.1.

Confidence Intervals

Confidence intervals are also essential to inferential statistical procedures. Whereas a hypothesis test examines the probability that a sample was drawn from a population with a single parameter, confidence intervals provide a range of values of the population parameter that are plausible given a set of data. The degree of confidence in the interval is based on the researcher's established Type I error rate. A Type I error rate set at 5% is associated with a 95% (100% − 5% = 95%) confidence interval. Two-sided confidence intervals consist of a lower and upper bound for plausible values of the true population. For example, a 95% confidence interval for a mean could be 10 to 20, and a researcher would interpret this as being 95% confident that the true population mean is between 10 and 20. This very simple example exemplifies how the confidence intervals provide more information about the population parameter of interest than testing against a null hypothesis. If a researcher were testing a null hypothesis that states that the mean is equal to 5 and rejecting this null hypothesis, then she is only left knowing what the population mean is not likely to equal. By calculating a confidence interval, then the researcher would know what range of population mean values were plausible given the data, in addition to knowing which values are unlikely. Given the amount of information yielded by confidence intervals, it is recommended that researchers report confidence intervals when reporting the results of hypothesis testing.

Confidence intervals also give researchers an idea about the precision based on the width of the interval. Confidence interval calculations are based on the sampling distribution of the statistic of interest. As presented earlier in this appendix, the standard deviation of the sampling distribution

TABLE A.1. Summary of Decisions in Hypothesis Testing

Decision	True state of nature	
	True null hypothesis	False null hypothesis
Reject null hypothesis	Type I error Probability = α	Correct decision Probability = $1 - \beta$ = power
Fail to reject null hypothesis	Correct decision Probability = $1 - \beta$	Type II error Probability = β

Note. Data from Sheskin (2007).

is called standard error. Thus, when standard errors are higher, then confidence intervals will be wider, or less precise. Recall that a large standard error indicates that there is more variability between samples of the same size drawn from a population. A large standard error suggests that there is a large amount of variation between members of the populations. It should be logical then that a confidence interval would be wider in this instance (i.e., a large standard error) because it would be more difficult to know where the true population parameter lies. Conversely, when a sampling distribution has a very small standard error, it suggests that each sample drawn from a population is fairly similar. As a result of the smaller standard error, the confidence interval will be narrower.

Effect Size

Given the dependency that exists between statistically significant findings and sample sizes, an additional measure should be included when reporting results of statistical analysis. The measure is referred to as an effect size and represents the magnitude of an effect in standardized units. As sample sizes increase, then statistical significance (i.e., $p < \alpha$) becomes more easily achieved. This phenomenon is true to the point where even very small deviations from the null hypothesis will be statistically significant when the sample size is very large. Effect sizes, in contrast, are calculated based on standard deviation units and are less heavily influenced by sample size. As a result, effect sizes are often thought of as representing practical significance.

There are many measures of effect size depending on a number of elements, such as sample statistic and analysis plan. The statistical analytic procedures presented in this appendix will be accompanied by Cohen's *d* index (Cohen, 1977, 1988). Cohen also provided guidelines to assist with the interpretation of various values of his *d* index. A value of *d* below 0.5 is a small effect, from 0.5 to 0.8 a medium effect, and greater than 0.8 a large effect. Values of *d* between 0.5 and 0.8 represent medium effects, and values greater than 0.8 indicate large effects. It should be noted that these guidelines were developed to assist with effect size interpretations on the whole. The convention might not hold across all cases, and the researcher should decide the appropriate levels of small, medium, and large effects based on his or her research context.

Inferential Procedures

In this section, four commonly used statistical procedures for comparing means will be presented. The discussion of each procedure will include the context in which the test would be conducted, assumptions, null hypotheses, standard errors, 95% confidence intervals, and effect sizes.

One-Sample *t*-Test

The one-sample *t*-test is used to determine whether or not a sample was derived from a population with a particular mean. The assumptions for the one-sample *t*-test are that the sample was randomly drawn from the population, the data are normally distributed, and the observations are not related to each other in any meaningful way; that is, the observations are independent. These assumptions must be assessed so as not to jeopardize the trustworthiness of the analysis.

An example will help illustrate this description. The provider of a new employee assistant program (EAP) markets its services to companies that want to improve their employees' well-being and job performance. The provider of the EAP claims that employees who use its services report higher levels of job satisfaction than the general workforce. As a part of the EAP, the provider develops a job satisfaction survey and collects responses from a sample of 50 employees who have used their EAP. The mean sum score for the survey scale is 34.4 points, with a standard deviation of 6 points. The EAP provider also claims that the national average for job satisfaction is 29 points. An interested but skeptical human resources (HR) director wants to test the EAP provider's claim that employees who use EAP services report higher levels of job satisfaction than the general workforce. The HR staff conducts a test to see if the mean of 34.4 is statistically higher than the national mean of 29. Note that because the statistical test seeks to determine not only if there is a difference in the means but also if the sample mean is *greater than* the reported population mean, the director must conduct a one-sided, directional hypothesis test.

Before moving into the hypothesis test, the assumptions of the one-sample *t*-test must be assessed. The first assumption is assessed not by statistics but rather by the research design. In this scenario, the responses to the job satisfaction instrument were reportedly selected at random. The EAP provider also reported that only one employee was sampled from each company, so no violations of independence were noted.

The assumption of normality can be assessed visually or by conducting a normality test. To assess the normality assumption visually, one could use histograms or quantile–quantile (Q–Q) plots. A histogram is like a visual representation of the frequency distribution discussed in Chapter 7. That is, the height of each bar, or bin, reflects the frequency of values that fall within the range values represented by each bar. This method of assessing the normality assumption is presented in Figure A.1. Using statistical software, a histogram was generated from the data collected, and a normal curve was overlaid to more easily see deviations from normality. The data do not perfectly follow the normal distribution, but the distribution does appear to be approximately normal. Thus, no violations of model assumptions are noted.

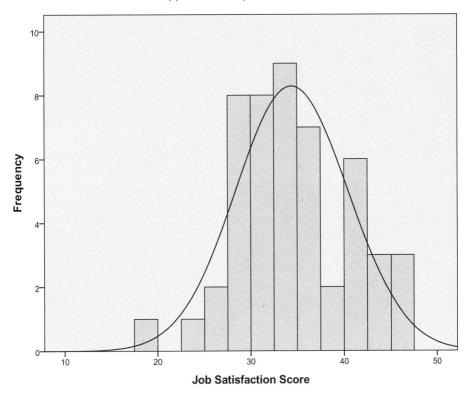

Job Satisfaction Score

FIGURE A.1. A histogram for assessing the normality assumption.

A Q–Q plot is a graphical technique for assessing the correspondence between two distributions. In this case, one of the distributions is the scores from the job satisfaction survey and the other distribution is a normal distribution. If the job satisfaction scores are normally distributed, the Q–Q plot should approximately form a straight line on a 45° angle. A straight line indicates direct correspondence between the distribution of scores and a normal distribution. The Q–Q plot is presented in Figure A.2.

In this scenario, the sample mean is 34.4 points and the population mean is 29 points. Thus, the HR director wishes to find the probability that the deviation between 34.4 and 29 is due to random chance, or the probability that the sample was drawn from a population with a mean different from 29 points. Previously, we stated that the null hypothesis represents chance occurrence of the sample statistic. Thus, the null hypothesis would be written as $H_0: \mu = 29$. This states that the true job satisfaction mean is 29, but the deviation that was observed was due to randomness, or luck of the draw. The one-sided, directional alternative hypothesis could be written as $H_1: \mu > 29$. This states that the sample was not drawn from

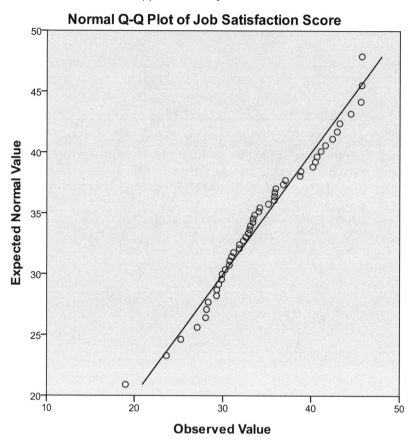

FIGURE A.2. A Q–Q plot for assessing the correspondence between two distributions.

a population where the mean is greater than 29. This determination will be made after comparing the deviation with the average amount of deviation between samples repeatedly drawn from the population (i.e., standard error). The HR director decided to use a Type I error rate of 5%.

The first step in this hypothesis test was already completed. That is, the sample mean and standard deviation must be calculated or computed. These types of calculations were described in Chapter 7, and they are commonly found using statistical software packages. In the current scenario, the sample mean is 34.4 with standard deviation of 6. Next, a test statistic is computed, which reflects the ratio of the observed deviation between sample mean and hypothesized population mean to the expected deviation in the sampling distribution (i.e., standard error). The formula for the test statistic in a one-sample *t*-test is

$$t = \frac{\bar{x} - \mu}{s_{\bar{x}}} = \frac{\bar{x} - \mu}{\dfrac{\hat{s}}{\sqrt{n}}} = \frac{34.4 - 29}{\dfrac{6}{\sqrt{50}}} = 6.35$$

The test statistic of $t = 6.35$ suggests that the deviation that was observed is slightly more than six times as much as the average amount of deviation between the means if samples of 50 people were repeatedly drawn from the population. The question that remains is if this difference is large enough to conclude that the sample statistic of 34.4 is significantly greater than the hypothesized population mean of 29. The statistician must then find the probability associated with a test statistic of 6.35 within the context of the study. The probability can be found using a statistical software package or a table of critical values that can be found in most statistics textbooks. In this text, statistical software will be used to carry out the one-sample t-test. The sample output is provided in Figure A.3.

One can see that the test statistic is presented in the "t" column, and the difference between the sample mean and the hypothesized population mean is found in the column labeled "Mean Difference." The "df" column shows the degrees of freedom for this t-test. In essence, degrees of freedom represent the total amount of information a researcher has in his or her dataset, where higher degrees of freedom imply more information is contained in the dataset. Degrees of freedom are calculated for the one-sample t-test by $df = n - 1$, where n is the number of participants in the study. The sample size in this test was 50, which means that we have 49 degrees of freedom.

We must stop here to discuss the implications of conducting a one-sided, directional hypothesis test. The statistical software output shown in this appendix is from SPSS, but SPSS does not provide one-sided tests. It

One-Sample Statistics

	N	Mean	Std. Deviation	Std. Error Mean
Job Satisfaction Score	50	34.41	6.020	.851

One-Sample Test

	Test Value = 29					
					95% Confidence Interval of the Difference	
	t	df	Sig. (2-tailed)	Mean Difference	Lower	Upper
Job Satisfaction Score	6.353	49	.000	5.409	3.70	7.12

FIGURE A.3. SPSS output for the one-sample t-test from the EAP job satisfaction improvement example.

is up to the user to make the appropriate adjustments to the output, which we outline below.

The column labeled "Sig. (2-tailed)" contains the probability of observing an absolute mean difference of 5.4 or greater if the null hypothesis were true. The probability is also called the p-value. In other words, this is a two-sided hypothesis p-value, and we are interested in the one-sided p-value. Therefore, we need to divide the p-value provided by SPSS by two because we only want a one-sided test. The probability appears to be equal to zero, but this is only due to rounding. The probability is actually equal to 3.3×10^{-8}, which is very small. This probability is compared against the preestablished Type I error rate of 5%. The one-sided p-value is less than .05, which allows the HR director to conclude with 95% confidence that the true mean in the population is greater than 29.

As mentioned previously, the researcher should also look at the 95% confidence interval to determine which values of the population mean are plausible. Again, SPSS provides the confidence interval for a two-sided test, so we need to make the appropriate adjustment once again. To provide the confidence interval for a one-sided test, we must perform our own calculations. We conducted a test to see if the population mean for the EAP users was *greater than* 29, which means we conducted an upper-tail test. Upper-tail tests are associated with finding the lower bound of the confidence interval. For this, we need three pieces of information: the sample mean, the standard error, and the one-sided critical value from the t distribution with 49 degrees of freedom. The sample mean is 34.4. The standard error is given by SPSS as 0.851. The critical value is 1.68, which we obtained from a table of critical values. The lower bound of the confidence interval is

$$CI_{LB} = 34.4 - (1.68 * 0.851) = 32.97$$

Therefore, the HR director can also conclude with 95% confidence that the true mean job satisfaction score of those employees who participated in the EAP is at least about 33 points.

Through the HR director's investigation, it was concluded that the EAP provider may have underreported the actual job satisfaction. However, one final decision remains for the HR professional. Is the difference between the reported mean job satisfaction of 29 points and the actual mean job satisfaction observed of 34.4 points a big enough difference for the company to enroll in the new EAP? An effect size estimate would likely aid in this decision-making process.

The formula for Cohen's d index for the one-sample t-test is $d = (\bar{x} - \mu)/\hat{s}$. Thus, the d index in this job satisfaction scenario is equal to $d = (34.4 - 29)/6 = 0.9$, which according to Cohen's (1988) convention is a large effect. Still, the company should consider this information in conjunction with whether 5.4 additional points above the EAP marketing assertions is worth investing in the EAP.

Dependent-Samples *t*-Test

The dependent-samples *t*-test, also known as the paired-samples *t*-test, matched-pairs *t*-test, or the *t*-test for related samples, is applied when comparing the means between groups that are not independent. For example, if a researcher were interested in examining the change before and after an intervention, then the samples would be dependent because they consist of exactly the same people. Another example could involve research based on data collected from siblings. The samples are not independent because siblings are likely to share many characteristics that could confound statistical analyses when treated as independent. Thus, the dependent-samples *t*-test recognizes the correlated nature of the data and adjusts the test statistic accordingly.

The assumptions for the test are (1) the data follow a normal distribution and (2) the observations within each sample are independent. The second assumption can be slightly confusing, but the *samples* are related, not *observations* within samples. Within each sample, there should be no relationships between members.

Suppose a school district hires an evaluator to examine the effect of an after-school program on self-esteem among middle school students. Self-esteem is to be measured by a 15-item scale from which responses will be summed to create a scale score. The evaluator also wants to mitigate the effect of academic achievement on self-esteem. Thus, he wants to match the students on the basis of academic achievement using grade point average (GPA). Fifty students are selected at random and matched by GPA, such that there are two samples of 25 matched pairs. One student in each of the pairs is randomly offered the opportunity to participate in the after-school program. The group of students who are participating in the after-school program will be referred to as the treatment group, and those not participating will be called the control group.

In the case of the dependent-samples *t*-test, the evaluator is interested in any differences that may exist between the pairs of students. Therefore, he wants to know if the mean difference on the self-esteem scale between the groups is different from zero, which provides him with the null hypothesis. The data referred to in the assumptions are the difference scores, and they should be normally (or nearly normally) distributed. This assumption can be checked in the same way as presented in the one-sample *t*-test discussion. The difference scores are calculated by simply subtracting the scores of one group from the other group within each pair. Subtracting the scores of the treatment group from the scores of the control group will result in exactly the same result as when the scores of the control group are subtracted from the scores of the treatment group.

Suppose the evaluator checks the assumption of normally distributed differences using a histogram and determines that the assumption is tenable. Next, he finds the difference in each pair by subtracting the control group member's score from the matched, treatment group member's score. Subsequently, he finds the average of the differences $(\bar{x}_d)$ is equal to 1.24, and the standard deviation of the differences is equal to 3.89. With this information, the evaluator can begin his hypothesis test, and he establishes the Type I error rate as 5%.

As stated before, the null hypothesis is that the true mean difference in the population is equal to zero $(H_0: \mu_D = 0)$. The null hypothesis in essence states that the after-school program has no effect on student's self-esteem, or that any differences observed between groups is purely due to chance. The nondirectional alternative hypothesis is that the mean difference in the population is not equal to zero. Note that this hypothesis does not specify if one group had higher self-esteem than the other; it only states that the groups' means are not equal.

The test statistic can be calculated using the following formula or computed with a statistical software package.

$$t = \frac{\bar{x}_d - \mu_0}{\frac{\hat{s}_d}{\sqrt{n}}} = \frac{1.24 - 0}{\frac{3.89}{\sqrt{25}}} = \frac{1.24}{0.777} = 1.595$$

The output from the statistical software is provided in Figure A.4.

The column labeled "Mean" contains the calculated mean difference, and the "Std. Deviation" column shows the standard deviation of the differences. The "Std. Error Mean" column contains the standard error of the mean, which is equal to 0.777 and is used as the denominator in the test statistic formula above. The 95% confidence interval columns are next, and the lower and upper bounds are equal to –0.36 and 2.84, respectively. This suggests that the evaluator can conclude with 95% confidence that the true difference in self-esteem in the population between students who do and do not participate in the after-school program is between –0.36 and 2.84. This raises an important point about confidence intervals. The reader will notice that the 95% confidence interval contains some values that favor one group (i.e., negative values) and some values that favor the other group (i.e., positive values). Thus, based on this information, the evaluator cannot be sure if the after-school program is effective in boosting self-esteem. Examining the p-value found in the "Sig. 2-tailed" column also tells the evaluator that he does not have sufficient evidence to reject the null hypothesis

Paired Samples Test

		Paired Differences							
					95% Confidence Interval of the Difference				
		Mean	Std. Deviation	Std. Error Mean	Lower	Upper	t	df	Sig. (2-tailed)
Pair 1	Treatment - Control	1.24000	3.88673	.77735	-.36436	2.84436	1.595	24	.124

FIGURE A.4. SPSS output for the dependent-samples t-test from the self-esteem example.

207

because the p-value ($p = .124$) is larger than the Type I error rate ($\alpha = .05$). The important point about confidence intervals is that if the value of the population parameter hypothesized under the null hypothesis is contained in the null hypothesis, then the p-value will not exceed the Type I error rate. In fact, the confidence interval contains all values for null hypotheses that would be retained by a hypothesis test. The degrees of freedom for this t-test are calculated by taking the number of pairs minus 1 ($df = n - 1$). Thus, this test has 24 degrees of freedom.

In this case, the evaluator determines that he cannot conclude that the after-school program is effective in changing students' self-esteem based on the evidence provided in the study. In order to report the effect size, Cohen's d index would be estimated using the following formula.

$$\hat{d} = \frac{|\hat{\mu}_1 - \hat{\mu}_2|}{\hat{s}_D} = \frac{|\hat{\mu}_D|}{\hat{s}_D} = \frac{1.24}{3.89} = 0.319$$

The difference between the group means on the original outcome variable metric is 1.24, as noted above. The difference between the group means on a standardized scale is 0.319, which is what the effect size reflects. In other words, the difference between the group means is about a third of a standard deviation. The guidelines for interpreting Cohen's d are the same as presented earlier. In standardized units, the after-school program yielded a small effect. However, the hypothesis test did not provide sufficient evidence to conclude with 95% confidence that the mean difference in self-esteem between the two groups was different from zero. Even in the event of statistically nonsignificant findings, the effect size should still be reported. This is because it is possible that the statistical test did not have sufficient power to detect the difference. The effect size could be used for calculating statistical power, but conducting power analysis after the fact is usually an effort in futility. For more information on using effect sizes to conduct post-hoc power analysis, see Cohen (1988).

Independent-Samples t-Test

As the name implies, the independent-samples t-test is used to compare the means between two groups that are independent of, or unrelated to, each other. Unlike the dependent-samples t-test, the groups in this test should be uncorrelated, and the members within each group should be uncorrelated. The sample means, denoted by $\bar{x}_1$ and $\bar{x}_2$, are used as estimates of the population means (μ_1 and μ_2) from which they are derived. The independent-samples t-test has three assumptions: (1) the samples were randomly selected from the populations they represent, (2) the data are normally distributed, and (3) the variances of the populations from which the samples were drawn are equal. The third assumption is also referred to as homogeneity of variance. Recall that in Chapter 7 we described the variance as the mean sum of the squared differences.

Consider the following example. The director of a teacher professional development program wants to conduct a program evaluation. One of the many outcomes is increased self-efficacy of teachers who complete the program. She randomly selects 10 teachers from her school district with three or fewer years of experience and offers them the opportunity to complete the program. They all agree to participate. At the conclusion of the program, the director administers a self-efficacy survey scale that has been shown to produce reliable information and support valid inferences. She also randomly selects 10 more teachers, who did not participate in the program, and requests that they complete the self-efficacy scale as well. For both groups of teachers, the sum score on the survey scale was used as an estimate of self-efficacy.

The sample mean and standard deviation for the group of teachers who participated in the professional development program are 38.6 ($\bar{x}_1$) and 8.3 ($\hat{s}_1$), respectively. The sample mean and standard deviation for the group of teachers who did not participate in the professional development program are 35.8 ($\bar{x}_2$) and 8.9 ($\hat{s}_2$). Clearly, the mean self-efficacy score was higher for the teachers who participated than for the teachers who did not, but the director wants to know if this difference is likely true among all new teachers. To make this determination, she will conduct a hypothesis test of these data using a Type I error rate of 5%.

With regard to assessing the tenability of the assumptions, the participants were randomly selected, and the director examined histograms, Q–Q plots, and normality tests to determine whether the data were approximately normally distributed. The homogeneity of variance assumption was tested using a separate hypothesis test, called Levene's test for homogeneity of variance, that can help researchers decide whether the variance of the scores in each group are equal. In the current example, the p-value for Levene's test ($p = .928$) was larger than the Type I error rate ($\alpha = .05$). Thus, she fails to reject the null hypothesis, which suggests that the assumption of equal variances has not been violated. The results of Levene's test of homogeneity of variance are provided by statistical software. For more information regarding Levene's test, see Levene (1960).

The null hypothesis in the independent-samples t-test states that the two population means are equal (H_0: $\mu_1 = \mu_2$ or $\mu_1 - \mu_2 = 0$). Because the true population means remain unknown, the sample means are used as estimates of the population means. The alternative hypothesis states that the population means are not equal (H_1: $\mu_1 \neq \mu_2$). Next, the test statistic must be calculated using the following formula.

$$t = \frac{(\bar{x}_1 - \bar{x}_2) - (\mu_1 - \mu_2)}{\sqrt{\dfrac{\hat{s}_1^2}{n_1} + \dfrac{\hat{s}_2^2}{n_2}}} = \frac{(38.6 - 35.8) - 0}{\sqrt{\dfrac{8.3^2}{10} + \dfrac{8.9^2}{10}}} = \frac{2.8}{3.856} = 0.726$$

The output from the statistical software is presented in Figure A.5.

The degrees of freedom for the independent-samples *t*-test are calculated by taking the overall sample size for both groups and subtracting 2: $df = (n_1 + n_2) - 2 = (10 + 10) - 2 = 18$. Two degrees of freedom were subtracted since the mean was calculated for each of the two groups. In the output, the value found in the column labeled "Mean Difference" is simply the difference when the Group 2 mean ($\bar{x}_2 = 35.8$) is subtracted from the Group 1 mean ($\bar{x}_1 = 38.6$). The standard error of the difference is 3.856, which is the denominator in the test statistic formula above. The 95% confidence interval columns show that the true difference between Group 1 and Group 2 is likely between –5.30 and 10.90 points. That is, the director can conclude with 95% confidence that the mean self-efficacy score for the teachers who participate is somewhere between 5.30 points *lower than* or 10.90 points *higher than* the mean self-efficacy score for teachers who do not participate in the program. One can see that the *p*-value in the column labeled "Sig. (2-tailed)" ($p = .477$) is greater than the Type I error rate of .05. Thus, the director does not have sufficient evidence to reject the null hypothesis that the group means are equal.

Statistical significance does not imply practical significance. The director should next calculate Cohen's *d* index to determine how meaningful the difference between group means is by examining the standardized difference in scores. The formula for the *d* index for independent samples is presented below. Note that the denominator is the pooled standard deviation. This is used because rarely are the standard deviations from both groups the same, and the pooled standard deviation combines the standard deviations from both groups into a weighted average.

$$\hat{d} = \frac{|\bar{x}_1 - \bar{x}_2|}{\hat{s}_{\text{pooled}}} = \frac{|\bar{x}_1 - \bar{x}_2|}{\sqrt{\dfrac{(n_1 - 1)\hat{s}_1^2 + (n_2 - 1)\hat{s}_2^2}{(n_1 + n_2) - 2}}}$$

$$= \frac{|38.6 - 35.8|}{\sqrt{\dfrac{(10 - 1)8.3^2 + (10 - 1)8.9^2}{(10 + 10) - 2}}} = \frac{|2.8|}{8.61} = 0.325$$

The effect size estimate of 0.325 is a small effect based on Cohen's convention of effect size classification for social sciences. In standardized units, the professional development program yielded a small effect,

Independent Samples Test

		Levene's Test for Equality of Variances		t-test for Equality of Means					95% Confidence Interval of the Difference	
		F	Sig.	t	df	Sig. (2-tailed)	Mean Difference	Std. Error Difference	Lower	Upper
VAR00002	Equal variances assumed	.008	.928	.726	18	.477	2.80000	3.85573	-5.30059	10.90059
	Equal variances not assumed			.726	17.913	.477	2.80000	3.85573	-5.30341	10.90341

FIGURE A.5. Sample SPSS output from the independent-samples t-test.

although the hypothesis test did not provide sufficient evidence to conclude with 95% confidence that the mean difference between group was different from zero.

One-Way Analysis of Variance

Analysis of variance (ANOVA) refers to a family of procedures first introduced by Sir Ronald Fisher that were used to evaluate whether a difference existed between at least two means in a dataset from which two or more means could be computed (Sheskin, 2007). That is, ANOVA can be used to compare group means when two or more groups are represented. In this section, the most basic ANOVA model will be presented. Also called the single-factor between-subjects ANOVA, this procedure is most commonly referred to as the one-way ANOVA model. In the previous section, we presented the independent-samples *t*-test, which is used to compare two groups. This test can only be used to compare two groups, whereas one-way ANOVA can be used whenever there are two or more groups. Thus, the independent-samples *t*-test can be viewed as a special case of one-way ANOVA because they are mathematically equivalent. Despite their equivalence, analysts typically employ the *t*-test when two groups are being compared and reserve one-way ANOVA for three or more groups. The assumptions of one-way ANOVA are the same as those of the independent-samples *t*-test: (1) each k sample is independent (where $k \geq 2$), (2) the data for each group are normally distributed, and (3) the variances for all groups are homogeneous. Violations of these assumptions may jeopardize the trustworthiness of the results.

For illustration, consider the following example. A manager of employee relations wanted to assess the views of diversity within the company to determine if there were differences between employees of different ethnic backgrounds. Using the employees' personnel records, he randomly selected 20 employees who had classified themselves into one of the company's four largest ethnic backgrounds: African American, Asian American, Caucasian, and Hispanic/Latino. The 80 employees were sent the company's previously validated perceptions of diversity survey scale, and their diversity scores were calculated by summing the responses to the 20-item scale. The means and standard deviations for employees in each ethnic group are presented in Table A.2.

Each employee was randomly sampled, which satisfies the first assumption. The manager screened the data for normality by conducting normality tests and examining the histograms, and no violations of normality were noted. To test the homogeneity of variance assumption, Levene's test was conducted using a Type I error rate of 5% against the null hypothesis that the variances across groups ($H_0: \sigma_1^2 = \sigma_2^2 = \sigma_3^2 = \sigma_4^2$). The results of this test are shown in Figure A.6. As can be seen by examining the "Sig." column,

TABLE A.2. Descriptive Statistics by Ethnic Group

Ethnicity	Mean	Standard deviation
African American	48.58	17.20
Asian American	38.30	8.71
Caucasian	40.05	11.26
Hispanic/Latino	56.56	16.98

the *p*-value is less than .05. Thus, the manager rejects the null hypothesis that the variances are equal, which indicates that the third assumption has been violated. The reader should note that this violation was presented intentionally because it occurs frequently in practice. A brief discussion of handling this violation is presented following the one-way ANOVA output.

The null hypothesis in one-way ANOVA states that all group means are equal (H_0: $\mu_1 = \mu_2 = \mu_3 = \mu_4$). Another way to interpret the null hypothesis is that all of the means were drawn from the same population. The alternative hypothesis, in contrast, states that at least one of the group means is different from at least one of the other group means (H_0: $\mu_k \neq \mu_{k'}$, where $k \neq k'$). The test statistic for the one-way ANOVA is the *F*-test statistic, and its calculation is more complex than that for the *t*-test statistic. The *F*-test statistic is based on finding the sums of squares between groups and the sums of squares within groups. Fortunately, these estimates are provided by the statistical software and are presented in both the following formula and Figure A.7.

$$F = \frac{MS_B}{MS_W} = \frac{1423.283}{195.959} = 7.263$$

The mean square between groups as shown in this formula is calculated by dividing the sum of squares by the between-group degrees of freedom. Thus, it can be taken as a kind of average distance between each group mean and the overall mean for the entire dataset (i.e., the grand

Test of Homogeneity of Variances

Diversity

Levene Statistic	df1	df2	Sig.
4.207	3	76	.008

FIGURE A.6. Sample SPSS output from Levene's test of the homogeneity of variance assumption.

ANOVA

Diversity

	Sum of Squares	df	Mean Square	F	Sig.
Between Groups	4269.850	3	1423.283	7.263	.000
Within Groups	14892.900	76	195.959		
Total	19162.750	79			

FIGURE A.7. ANOVA output for diversity example.

mean). The mean square within group is the within-group sum of squares divided by the within-group degrees of freedom. The mean square within group can be interpreted as the average distance between an individual person's score and her group's mean. Had all of the assumptions been met, the test statistic would be equal to 7.263, and its associated p-value is less than .001. However, the homogeneity of variance assumption was violated, which means adjustments must be made to correct for the violated assumption.

Welch's (1951) adjustment can be applied in the event of violated homogeneity of variance assumption. In essence, Welch's test adjusts the degrees of freedom so that the results are robust against the violation. This test, too, is provided by the statistical software, and the results of Welch's test are presented in Figure A.8.

The test statistic is slightly lower in Welch's test, but the decision regarding the null hypothesis remains the same: At least one of the means differs from the other group means. The question then is which one(s)? Post-hoc analysis can help the manager answer this question. One such post-hoc analysis is Tukey's honestly significant difference (HSD) test. Tukey post-hoc analysis makes all pairwise comparisons. That is, it compares each group mean to every other group mean, and it does so without inflating the Type I error rate. The output from Tukey analysis in the diversity example is presented in Figure A.9.

Robust Tests of Equality of Means

Diversity

	Statistic[a]	df1	df2	Sig.
Welch	7.037	3	40.734	.001

a. Asymptotically F distributed.

FIGURE A.8. Sample SPSS output of ANOVA using Welch adjustment.

Multiple Comparisons

Dependent Variable: Diversity

Tukey HSD

(I) Group	(J) Group	Mean Difference (I-J)	Std. Error	Sig.	95% Confidence Interval	
					Lower Bound	Upper Bound
1.00	2.00	10.25000	4.42673	.104	-1.3781	21.8781
	3.00	8.50000	4.42673	.228	-3.1281	20.1281
	4.00	-8.05000	4.42673	.273	-19.6781	3.5781
2.00	1.00	-10.25000	4.42673	.104	-21.8781	1.3781
	3.00	-1.75000	4.42673	.979	-13.3781	9.8781
	4.00	-18.30000*	4.42673	.001	-29.9281	-6.6719
3.00	1.00	-8.50000	4.42673	.228	-20.1281	3.1281
	2.00	1.75000	4.42673	.979	-9.8781	13.3781
	4.00	-16.55000*	4.42673	.002	-28.1781	-4.9219
4.00	1.00	8.05000	4.42673	.273	-3.5781	19.6781
	2.00	18.30000*	4.42673	.001	6.6719	29.9281
	3.00	16.55000*	4.42673	.002	4.9219	28.1781

*. The mean difference is significant at the 0.05 level.

FIGURE A.9. SPSS results from the Tukey HSD test.

A glance down the column labeled "Sig." will reveal where the significant differences are between groups. The first p-value that is less than .05 is the comparison of Group 2 (Asian American) to Group 4 (Hispanic/Latino). The negative mean difference indicates that the mean diversity scale scores for the Hispanic/Latino employees is higher than that of the Asian American employees. Similarly, the comparison between Group 3 (Caucasian) and Group 4 (Hispanic/Latino) is statistically significant. The negative mean difference indicates that the mean diversity scale scores for the Hispanic/Latino employees is higher than that of the Caucasian employees.

In order to calculate the effect size for the one-way ANOVA, it is recommended that the d index be calculated for significant pairwise comparisons. In the diversity example, the manager would use the formula for the d index presented in the section on the independent-samples t-test. However, the pooled standard deviation should be taken from the ANOVA output. The pooled standard deviation is equal to the root mean square within group. To illustrate the calculation again, Cohen's d index is calculated for the comparison between Hispanic/Latino employees and Asian American employees.

$$d = \frac{|\bar{x}_1 - \bar{x}_2|}{\hat{s}_{pooled}} = \frac{|\bar{x}_1 - \bar{x}_2|}{\sqrt{MS_W}} = \frac{|38.3 - 56.6|}{13.999} = 1.307$$

The employee relations manager is able to conclude with 95% confidence that the mean diversity scale scores are not equal across ethnic groups. Post-hoc analysis revealed that Hispanic/Latino employees had higher scale scores than did Asian American and Caucasian employees. The d index for each of the significant comparisons was 1.307 and 1.182, respectively. Each of these values of the d index suggests a large effect.

Nonparametric Inferential Statistics

As stated previously, conducting hypothesis tests on group means requires that certain assumptions be met about the distribution(s). The preceding sections provide some guidelines for assessing the model assumptions and even offer steps for requesting adjusted output in the case of violations to the homogeneity of variance assumption. Although these adjustments will be helpful in many cases, researchers and program evaluators might also find themselves possessing data with non-normal distributions or data collected from small samples, which are less likely to satisfy the model assumptions. Fortunately, there is another branch of inferential statistics that can handle data with such challenges. This branch of procedures is called nonparametric inferential statistics, which is characterized by reduction or, in some cases, freedom from assumptions. In this section, we present two useful nonparametric procedures. These procedures are the analogs of the independent-samples t-test (i.e., the Mann–Whitney U test) and the one-way analysis of variance (i.e., the Kruskal–Wallis test).

Mann–Whitney *U* Test

The Mann–Whitney U test uses rank-order data in hypothesis testing scenarios with two independent samples. Researchers might collect rank-order data, or they can also transform their existing data into rank-order form. In the latter case, the non-normal data are transformed to have a different distribution; however, the data maintain the same rank order. The transformation of the data to rank-order data provides the basis for how the procedure deals with non-normally distributed data. By transforming the data, the researcher sacrifices information but might stand to gain statistical power. The Mann–Whitney test assumes that (1) the measurement scale is at least ordinal; (2) each sample was randomly selected from the population it represents; (3) observations are independent within and between samples; and (4) the distributions have the same shape. With these assumptions, the Mann–Whitney procedure can be used to test the group medians. The null hypothesis states that the group medians are equal (H_0: $\theta_1 = \theta_2$), and the nondirectional alternative hypothesis states that the group medians are unequal (H_1: $\theta_1 \neq \theta_2$). The directional alternative hypothesis states that one group median is greater or less than the other group median.

Computation of the test statistic is more complex than that for the independent-samples t-test and is complicated with the presence of tied ranks. Consider the data provided in the previous independent-samples t-test. First, the values from the overall sample must be ranked where the lowest value is ranked as 1. Ranks based on the independent-samples t-test data are presented in Table A.3. The lowest value in the entire set of data is 19, so it was assigned a rank of 1. The highest value in the set of data is 53, so it was assigned a rank of 20. Notice that when two values are equal to each other, or tied, the average of the ranks is used. For example, the value of 37 points appears twice in the sample, and these two values represent the 11th and 12th data points in the ordered set. Therefore, the average of these ranks, 11.5, is used as the rank for both.

The test statistic for the Mann–Whitney U test is then calculated using the following formula (from Sheskin, 2007).

$$U = n_1 n_2 + \frac{n_1(n_1 + 1)}{2} - \Sigma R_1$$

TABLE A.3. Rank Transformed Data

Group member	Participant group raw data	Nonparticipant group raw data	Participant group rank data	Nonparticipant group rank data
1	32	43	5	15
2	53	40	20	14
3	37	46	11.5	16
4	48	30	18.5	4
5	35	36	8.5	10
6	27	19	3	1
7	38	34	13	7
8	48	37	18.5	11.5
9	35	26	8.5	2
10	33	47	6	17
			$\Sigma = 112.5$	$\Sigma = 97.5$

where n_1 is the number of cases in the group with fewer people, n_2 is the number of cases in the group with more people, and ΣR_1 is the sum of the ranks in the group with fewer people. In the current example, each group consists of 10 people. Therefore, we will need to compute U for both groups and use the smaller of the values for the test statistic. Using the data provided in this example, we can calculate the test statistic for U_1 and U_2 as shown in the following equation.

$$U_1 = n_1 n_2 + \frac{n_1(n_1 + 1)}{2} - \Sigma R_1 = (10)(10) + \frac{10(10+1)}{2} - 112.5 = 42.5$$

$$U_2 = n_1 n_2 + \frac{n_2(n_2 + 1)}{2} - \Sigma R_2 = (10)(10) + \frac{10(10+1)}{2} - 97.5 = 57.5$$

In this example, $U_1 = 42.5$ and $U_2 = 57.5$, so we will use 42.5 for U because it is the smaller of U_1 and U_2.

In nonparametric statistics, many procedures perform an exact test, including Mann–Whitney. Unlike scenarios with continuous data, when ranks are used, there are a limited number of combinations that a fixed number of ranks can take. Each combination of possible observations is referred to as a permutation. In this scenario, one possible permutation is that all 10 of the teachers with the highest reported self-efficacy are in the first group. A second possible permutation is that the nine teachers with the highest reported self-efficacy and the teacher with the lowest reported self-efficacy are in the first group. A third possible permutation is that all 10 of the teachers with the lowest reported self-efficacy are in the first group and so on. Despite the number of permutations, we are able to find the exact probability of the permutation we observed as well as those that are less probable. This comprises the rejection region for the null hypothesis. However, the number of permutations increases very quickly as the number of cases increases. In the self-efficacy example, there are 184,756 unique combinations! Needless to say, computers are necessary to quickly find the probabilities associated with certain permutations.

Most statistics textbooks contain a table of values to determine whether to reject the null hypothesis. In the self-efficacy scenario, the critical value for the Mann–Whitney U test for two independent groups each containing 10 members and a Type I error rate of 5% is 23. In fact, this will be the critical value for any Mann–Whitney test that involves two groups of 10 people. Because we took the minimum value of U above, we are looking to see if our observed U value is less than the critical value. That is, any value of U less than 23 will result in a rejection of the null hypothesis that the medians for each group are equal. The calculated test statistic of 42 is greater than 23, so we cannot reject the null hypothesis with 95% confidence.

Although computers enable researchers to conduct exact tests, often approximations provide a sufficiently close alternative to exact tests, and they are much less processor intensive. In fact, many statistical software packages provide statistical output based on approximations. Figure A.10 presents the computer output for the Mann–Whitney U test using the self-efficacy data. Note that the U statistic is the same as calculated above (i.e., $U = 42.5$). The row that contains the Z value of $-.568$ is the test statistic for an approximation. Similarly, the row labeled "Asymp. Sig. (2-tailed)" shows the p-value associated with the approximate Z test statistic. The exact p-value is also provided, but the software did not correct for ties in the data. Thus, both p-values reported here are approximate, and both are much larger than the Type I error rate of 5%. Therefore, the researcher cannot conclude with 95% confidence that the medians are not equal. For more in-depth discussion of the Mann–Whitney U test, see Marascuilo and McSweeney (1977), Conover (1999), and Sheskin (2007).

Kruskal–Wallis One-Way Analysis of Variance

Just as the one-way analysis of variance was an extension of the independent-samples t-test, the Kruskal–Wallis one-way analysis of variance is an extension of the Mann–Whitney U test. That is, the Kruskal–Wallis one-way analysis of variance is capable of analyzing two or more groups. As such, it is also used to analyze the ranks of the raw data. The assumptions of the Kruskal–Wallis test are as follows:

1. The measurement scale is at least ordinal.
2. Each sample was randomly selected from the population it represents.

Test Statistics[a]

	VAR00002
Mann-Whitney U	42.500
Wilcoxon W	97.500
Z	-.568
Asymp. Sig. (2-tailed)	.570
Exact Sig. [2*(1-tailed Sig.)]	.579[b]

a. Grouping Variable: GROUP

b. Not corrected for ties.

FIGURE A.10. SPSS output for the Mann–Whitney U test.

3. Independence is met for within and between samples.

4. The distributions have the same shape.

The null hypothesis states that the medians of each k independent group are equal (H_0: $\theta_1 = \theta_2 = \ldots = \theta_k$). The alternative hypothesis states that at least two of the medians are not equal. The test statistic for the Kruskal–Wallis test is calculated using ranked data and procedures associated with the traditional ANOVA. First, the data should be ranked, assigning a rank of 1 to the lowest value in an entire sample of data collected. Next, the traditional ANOVA described earlier should be conducted using the ranks *instead of* the raw data.

Consider an illustration using a smaller dataset than was presented with the traditional one-way ANOVA. A researcher at a large organization was asked by a senior executive to investigate whether there is a difference in the ratings of middle-level managers by their subordinates. In particular, she was interested in knowing if there were differences on the basis of where the middle-level managers received their education (i.e., Ivy League institutions, private institutions, or state-supported institutions of higher education). The researcher randomly selected six subordinates of each manager to complete a manager rating scale. Each of the subordinates selected was drawn from different offices so as not to violate the assumption of independence. The manager rating scale yields a score based on 15 survey scale items ranging from 15 to 60. The data are presented in Table A.4.

TABLE A.4. Results of the Manager Rating Scale for Three Groups

Member	Ivy League[a]		Private		Public	
	Raw	Rank	Raw	Rank	Raw	Rank
1	30	5	43	10	26	3
2	38	7	57	16.5	51	13
3	49	12	42	8.5	52	14
4	48	11	25	2	57	16.5
5	60	18	42	8.5	54	15
6	36	6	29	4	17	1

[a]Brown University, Columbia University, Cornell University, Dartmouth College, Harvard University, Princeton University, the University of Pennsylvania, or Yale University.

The statistic for the Kruskal–Wallis analysis of variance is

$$H = \frac{(N-1)SS_B}{SS_T}$$

where N is the total sample size, SS_B is the between-groups sum of squares, and SS_T is the total sum of squares from the ANOVA output using the ranks. The ANOVA table based on the ranked data is shown in Figure A.11.

Using the appropriate pieces of information from the ANOVA table, we find that the test statistic for the manager example is 0.53.

$$H = \frac{(N-1)SS_B}{SS_T} = \frac{(18-1)(15.083)}{483.5} = 0.53$$

Most statistical software packages do not provide the exact test output for the k independent-samples Kruskal–Wallis analysis of variance, but Meyer and Seaman (2008) identified the critical values of the test statistic H for three- and four-group scenarios up to 35 cases per group. For a scenario with three groups and six cases per group, the critical value associated with a Type I error rate of 5% is 5.719. The test statistic calculated in the manager rating data of 0.53 does not exceed the critical value. This suggests that the executive does not have sufficient evidence to reject the null hypothesis of no differences in the ratings of managers by their subordinates on the basis of where the middle-level managers received their education.

In scenarios where the number of groups or number of cases per group exceed those provided by Meyer and Seaman (2008), approximations can be used. Although it is unnecessary for the manager rating data, the output based on approximations from the statistical software is provided below for illustration purposes. For the approximate test, chi-square is used as the

ANOVA

Rank

	Sum of Squares	df	Mean Square	F	Sig.
Between Groups	15.083	2	7.542	.242	.788
Within Groups	468.417	15	31.228		
Total	483.500	17			

FIGURE A.11. SPSS output for the analysis of variance for estimation of variance components used in calculation of the Kruskal–Wallis ANOVA test statistic.

Test Statistics[a,b]

	Rating
Chi-Square	.530
df	2
Asymp. Sig.	.767

a. Kruskal Wallis Test

b. Grouping Variable:

SchoolType

FIGURE A.12. SPSS output for the approximate Kruskal–Wallis, which is based on the χ^2 distribution.

test statistic with $k - 1$ degrees of freedom. With a p-value of .767 as shown in Figure A.12, again the researcher does not have sufficient evidence to reject the null hypothesis. Post-hoc or pairwise comparisons are possible using rank-based contrasts. For more information on these procedures, see Marascuilo and McSweeney (1977) and Conover (1999).

In this appendix, we examined the use of inferential statistics to take information about a sample and make inferences about, or generalizations to, the larger group. We also discussed parametric and nonparametric analyses appropriate for use with survey scale data.

FURTHER READING

Agresti, A., & Finlay, B. (2008). *Statistical methods for the social sciences* (4th ed.). Upper Saddle River, NJ: Prentice Hall.

> *Provides detailed discussions of inferential statistics. Offers numerous examples.*

Kirk, R. E. (2008). *Statistics: An introduction* (5th ed.). Belmont, CA: Thomson.

> *Provides detailed discussions of inferential statistics. Offers numerous examples.*

Salkind, N. J. (2012). *Statistics for people who (think they) hate statistics* (5th ed.). Thousand Oaks, CA: Sage.

> *Provides detailed discussions of inferential statistics. Offers numerous examples. This text is very readable for beginners.*

APPENDIX EXERCISES

1. What are the major differences between the purposes and uses of descriptive versus inferential procedures?

2. If you had to rely *only* on descriptive statistics or inferential statistics, which would you choose? Why?

3. Provide scenarios in which you might use a one-sample *t*-test, a dependent-samples *t*-test, an independent-samples *t*-test, and an analysis of variance.

Glossary of Key Terms

Acquiescence	Source of error in responses in which survey participants tend to select the positive option (e.g., "Agree," "True") regardless of the content of the items.
Alternative hypothesis	Rival hypothesis of the null hypothesis. Specifies how the null hypothesis is false. Denoted as H_1.
Closed-response items	Statements or questions that provide answer options from which the survey participant selects a response. Includes Likert-style items, checklists, and true–false variations.
Components	Attributes of a construct.
Concept	Observable phenomena, categories, or classes of objects. Concepts allow us to associate similar entities.
Conceptual framework	Narrative and a model that define the constructs in a study and specify a set of propositions that make explicit the relationships between those constructs.
Confidence intervals	A range of values of the population parameter that are plausible given a set of data.

225

Construct	Abstract concepts that are not directly observable. An attribute, trait, or characteristic expressed in an abstract manner.
Correlate	How one variable changes as another variable changes. The degree to which variables covary or change together.
Correlation coefficient	A statistic that can take any value from −1 to +1. Provides information about the nature of the relationship between variables. This information includes direction and strength.
Covary	A variable changes in correlation with another related variable, in a manner that might be predictive.
Data	Quantitative or verbal information.
Dependent variable	A variable that is affected by an independent variable.
Dimensions	Attributes of a construct.
Domains	Interrelated attributes that make up a construct and are measured by a survey scale.
Effect size	A representation of the magnitude of an effect in standardized units; an indicator of practical significance.
Eigenvalue	The amount of variation explained by a factor.
Exploratory factor analysis	A family of statistical procedures for reducing a set of variables (items) to derive a smaller set of new variables referred to as factors.
Factor	A variable that is an expression of a construct.
Factor loading	A type of measure that expresses the strength of the relationship between an item and each factor.
Field test	Administration of an instrument to provide data to examine its functioning; more extensive than a pilot test.
Hypothesis	An empirically testable statement that certain variables are related as proposed by a theory.

Independent variable	A variable that affects another variable.
Indicators	Behaviors or responses used as a measure of a construct.
Internal consistency	Estimate of reliability based on the correlations between items.
Item response scales (options)	Numerical scales (e.g., 1–4 or 1–6) and/or response labels (e.g., "Strongly disagree," "Disagree," "Agree," "Strongly agree").
Latent variable	An unobservable ability, attribute, or characteristic. (*See also* Construct.)
Mean	A measure of central tendency that involves summing scores and dividing by the number of scores.
Median	The value that separates scores into the upper 50% of scores and lower 50% of scores; the middle value in an ordered set of values.
Mode	Most frequent data point or value associated with a given variable.
Model	Diagram that provides a visual representation of a conceptual framework.
Multidimensional	A set of items that measure more than one factor (i.e., construct).
Narrative	Text that describes the research questions and the concepts associated with the research focus.
Null hypothesis	Statement that there is no effect of an independent variable (e.g., treatment, intervention).
Open-response items	Statements or questions that require a survey participant to form his or her answer.
Operational	Actual use of an instrument for data collection after initial development is completed.
Operationalize	Translate a construct into language (e.g., items) that allows the researcher to observe and measure attributes that represent the construct.

Parallel forms	Reliability estimate based on scores from two forms of an instrument with the same content, means, and standard deviation.
Parameters	Numerical values used to describe populations.
Phenomenon	An observable occurrence, event, process, activity, or program that is the focus of inquiry (i.e., a research study).
Pilot test	Administration of an instrument to examine such aspects as instructions, item formats, and item response options.
Population	All subjects or members of a group who share one or more characteristics of research interest.
Primacy effect	Tendency of respondents to select the option presented first when items are presented in a visual format.
Principal axis factoring	See Exploratory factor analysis.
Propositions	Statements that define and describe concepts or state the relationship between the concepts in a framework. The statements may take the form of a hypothesis.
Protocol	Procedures to be followed in data collection.
Questionnaire	Printed set of items used for data collection.
Random sampling	Sampling process in which every member of a population has a random chance of being selected.
Range	The difference between the lowest numerical value and highest value of a variable.
Raw score	Total value of responses from a survey participant.
Recency effect	Tendency of respondents to select the option presented last when items are presented in an auditory format.
Reliability	The degree to which respondents' scores are consistent.

Response scale	The numerical or verbal component of a closed-response item where a survey participant records his or her answer.
Sample	Subsets of subjects or members who are selected from a population.
Scale scores	Scores formed by transforming raw scores to have a given mean and standard deviation.
Scatterplot	A plot containing the values of two variables.
Score stability	Reliability of scores across occasions.
Scree plot	A plot of the eigenvalues with the number of factors listed along the x-axis and the eigenvalue (i.e., the amount of variation explained by each factor) on the y-axis.
Standard deviation	Represents the typical distance of a value in a distribution from the sample mean.
Standard error	Reflects how far each sample mean is away from the expected population mean given the sample size. Standard deviation of the sampling distribution.
Statistics	Numerical values used to describe samples; considered estimates of population parameters.
Subscales	Components of a scale; operational form of the components of a construct.
Survey	A data-collection instrument that could include open- and closed-response items.
Survey scale	Instrument composed of closed-response items; measures a construct. It is the operational form of a construct.
Theory	A unified system of interrelated constructs, definitions, and propositions that describe a systematic view of phenomena with the purpose of explaining and predicting the phenomena.
Trait	An ability, attribute, or characteristic.

Unidimensional	A set of items that measure one factor (i.e., construct).
Validity	The degree to which evidence and theory support interpretation of scores for a given use of an instrument.
Variables	Constructs that have been operationalized. Variables can be measured and vary among survey participants. Independent variables are theorized to influence outcome variables (i.e., dependent variables).
Variance	The mean of the squared deviation scores where a deviation score is the difference between a single score and the mean for a distribution.

Sample Solutions to Chapter Exercises

CHAPTER 1

1. There are many possible answers to this item. A survey that one of the authors recently completed was developed by one of his students to measure medical care provider comfort when providing services to children with autism. He completed the instrument as an expert reviewer rather than a member of the intended target population. Regardless, the purpose of the survey was to measure the comfort of doctors who are performing check-ups on children with autism. The items on the survey focused on such areas as familiarity with medical conditions often associated with autism, confidence in one's ability to communicate with a patient with autism, comfort in one's ability to calm a patient with autism who is in distress, and ability to identify environmental triggers that may lead to sensory overload for a patient with autism.

2. The items in Figure 1.4 use a Likert-type response scale. Therefore, they can be classified as Likert-style items.

3. The items in Figure 1.4 provide response options from which each respondent may select one. Thus, the items are closed-response.

4. There are many possible answers to this prompt. A few additional statements for the Academic Engagement subscale are:

    . . . participate in class discussions.
    . . . read assigned readings before coming to class.
    . . . rarely pay attention to my teacher.

5. There are many possible answers to this prompt. A few additional statements for the Social Engagement subscale are:

. . . participate in extracurricular activities.

. . . have an interest in student government.

. . . come to school primarily to spend time with friends.

   a. The items focus on different aspects of engagement (Academic vs. Social).

   b. The items are formatted similarly and are conceptually similar to other items in their respective subscale.

6. It is primarily an issue of validity because the addition of an interpersonal relationships subscale may provide a more comprehensive representation of the important factors related to successful student transition.

CHAPTER 2

1. Validity refers to the accuracy of inferences based on information provided by an instrument. It is always important to ensure appropriate alignment between the target phenomenon and the instrument, and clarifying the purpose of the instrument may help researchers provide a stronger connection between the instrument and the target phenomenon.

2. The review of journal articles and professional critiques of the instrument will deepen one's understanding of other scholars' conceptualizations of the construct. In those outlets, readers will be able to read about specific uses and results of data collected from various samples. Taken together, one may develop a more comprehensive understanding of how others have used an existing instrument as well as under which circumstances the instrument yields useful data.

3.

Content Evaluation	Notes	Acceptable	Not Acceptable
1. Publisher's description and rationale for including the items in the instrument.	*The review provides information about the theoretical foundation and six understandings of human behavior.*	✓	
2. Quality of the items.	*The actual items are not included in the review, but reliability and validity evidence was provided. The authors included teacher focus groups for item generation. The internal consistency estimates were acceptable, but test–retest reliability was a little low.*	✓	
3. Currency of the content measured by the items on the instrument.	*Teacher focus groups were involved in the creation, which likely supports the currency of content included in the instrument.*	✓	

| 4. Match of the content of the instrument items to the evaluation or the research focus. | *The review provides information about the theoretical foundation and six understandings of human behavior.* | ✓ | |
| 5. The extent to which the items are inclusive and attend to diversity. | *It is not clear from the review the extent to which the items are inclusive and attend to diversity. The norm sample did include teachers from special education classrooms, but this is only one of many areas of diversity to which items could attend.* | | ✓ |

4. The reported estimates for internal consistency were that they "exceeded .90," which is within the range of acceptable reliability coefficients. The reported test–retest coefficients ranged from .30 to .70, which are low overall. Estimates equal to .70 may be acceptable for some purposes, but coefficients lower than .70 are not accepted by most fields.

5. We would consider adopting the Index of Teacher Stress instrument but would heed the cautions of Murray-Ward. We agree that the theoretical foundation and research base check out, but we would use it in conjunction with other important measures and data sources.

6. The MMY differs from the *Test Collection at ETS* in that the MMY also provides reviews and commentary of existing measures by respected scholars in the field. Both resources may be helpful in identifying existing instruments for potential adoption or adaptation.

7. One important difference between plagiarism and copyright infringement is that plagiarism is a matter of ethics and copyright infringement is a matter of the law. Plagiarism occurs when an author presents the words or ideas of another author as if the work were his or her own original work. Although plagiarism is extremely unethical, it is not illegal unless the plagiarized work is protected by copyright. Copyright infringement is the infringement on the rights of a copyright holder, which is illegal. Under copyright law, a work may not be used without permission.

CHAPTER 3

1. Student attitudes could be included as a variable for the "6. Student Outcomes" component in the conceptual framework.

2. In a job satisfaction survey, the Supervisory Relationship and Job Environment subscales may be considered independent, or explanatory, variables in a model where job satisfaction is the dependent, or outcome, variable. Those two variables can and have been theorized to be contributing factors to one's overall job satisfaction. Therefore, in a model that includes Supervisory Relationship, Job Environment, and Job Satisfaction, one would likely draw an arrow pointing from Supervisory Relationships or Job Environment to Job Satisfaction.

3. In our sample responses to a previous chapter's questions, we mentioned an instrument being developed to measure the comfortability of medical care providers when providing services (e.g., performing a physical examination) to patients with autism. In such cases, the quality of care may indeed be influenced by the medical providers' experience, familiarity, and/or knowledge of behaviors of patients with autism, all of which contribute to the care provider's comfort levels. The independent variable in this instance would be the care provider's comfort level, and the dependent variable would be the quality of care.

4. A conceptual framework may be used to connect the major components of a research or evaluation project to an integrated network of relationships. Not only does the framework assist the researcher with making sure that all important components are included, but it also is very useful to have the framework in a graphical or visual format. After the framework has been developed, it becomes a roadmap of sorts for making certain that measures (e.g., items or entire subscales) have been included to provide information about each of the important components.

CHAPTER 4

1. There are a few potential revisions to the item. First, terminology such as "instructional activities" may not be familiar to students responding to the item. Simplification of the language may be beneficial. Second, there are multiple ideas expressed in the item. The item may be broken into multiple items asked about each of the instructional activities individually. The response scale is not provided in the example, but a frequency response scale may be considered. Third, and related to the second point, the scale developer should include each of the instructional activities that are important to the purposes of the survey.

2. The phrase "special-needs students" should at least be revised to read "students with special needs" or possibly even "students with diverse learning needs."

3. The Flesch Reading Ease measure is 41.8, and the Flesch–Kincaid Grade Level is 10.1. The appropriateness of this reading level depends on the intended target audience. For employees with limited reading skills, the reading level may be too high. Lower reading levels are unlikely to influence respondents with high reading skills; so it would be wise to use simpler language in general.

4.

🚫 NOT THIS
During high school, I have been informed about the different opportunities available to receive college credit for classes taken while in high school (articulated credit, dual enrollment, concurrent enrollment).

✓ BUT THIS
I have been informed about the opportunities available to receive . . .

articulated credit.	Strongly disagree	Disagree	Agree	Strongly agree

| credit for dual enrollment. | Strongly disagree | Disagree | Agree | Strongly agree |
| credit for concurrent enrollment. | Strongly disagree | Disagree | Agree | Strongly agree |

Note to readers: We acknowledge that the revised item stems include specialized language; however, these items were used for the evaluation of a program for which awareness of this program-specific language was important.

CHAPTER 5

1. The prompt states that we want to know the activities in which socially engaged students participate. The prompt does **not** state that we are interested in frequency of participation in the provided activities. Therefore, a checklist would provide us with the information requested in the prompt. This would allow student respondents to simply place a checkmark by the activities in which they participate.

2. The response scale shown in an example of a Likert-type response scale.

3. a. First, the response scale does not seem appropriate for the item. Either the respondent goes to the gym weekly or not; it is not a statement with which there is likely to be degrees of agreement/disagreement. A potential revision is to revise the stem to read: How frequently do you visit the fitness gym? The possible response options could then be Daily, Weekly, Monthly, Never (see example below), or some such scale.

How frequently do you visit the fitness gym?	Never	Monthly	Weekly	Daily
	1	2	3	4

b. The response scale should be balanced. The difference between "Very Good" and "Excellent" is likely to be inconsequential for the purposes of the survey. The response option of "Very Good" could be deleted, and the response of "Excellent" would be worth 4 points instead of 5. There would be no fifth option (see example below).

Ease of making appointment through our website.	Poor	Fair	Good	Excellent
	1	2	3	4

We recommend formatting nonsubstantive response options apart from the substantive response options. In the case of 3c, if the "Do not know" option is necessary, then it should be removed from the middle of the scale and be presented by itself to the right of the agreement options (see the following example).

| c. | Students receive a more advanced learning experience at the Center for Knowledge than they would at their regularly assigned schools. | Disagree strongly ○ | Disagree ○ | Agree ○ | Agree strongly ○ | Do not know ○ |

CHAPTER 6

1. Although paper-and-pencil or web-based formats could be used to administer a survey that contained multiple Likert-type scales, the use of a web-based application would likely benefit the researcher most. With an online administration format, the researcher could format exactly how the items are shown whether it be one item on screen at a time or possibly one entire subscale on screen at a time. Data entry is also much easier with a web-based application because most current online survey services allow users to simply download the responses in a variety of file formats. Of course, it should be mentioned that the target respondents' access to technology should be carefully considered so as not to introduce response bias by only those who have access. Furthermore, when the researcher has direct access to respondents, as is sometimes the case when collecting data in schools or at academic conferences, a paper-based format can prove useful.

2. Suppose researcher A develops a survey to be administered online, and she generates one link that she will send to all members of her target sample. The same web link will be used by all respondents, and no identifying information will be collected on the survey. The responses collected in such a scenario can be considered anonymous because the researcher has no way to link a respondent's identification to any set of responses even if she wanted to. Now suppose researcher B develops a survey to be administered online, and he generates a unique link for each potential respondent. After each respondent uses his or her unique link to access the survey, the researcher will know which set of responses belong to which respondent. Yet, researcher B does not report the identifying information of any respondent. The responses collected in this scenario can be considered confidential because the researcher does know the identification of the respondents, but he will not report the information. The decision to collect personally identifying information should be determined by the plan for analysis of the data. For example, if the survey responses need to be linked with some other, existing dataset, then the researcher may need to collect identifying information so that she or he can link the data.

3. The use of eighth graders may yield *some* useful information, but this will depend on the degree of similarity between the 10 eighth graders and general ninth graders. In all likelihood, the eighth graders will not represent the views of ninth graders in general. On average, eighth and ninth graders are about 13–15 years old, which tends to be time of volatility in adolescent development; so one should carefully consider whether responses in eighth grade are likely to be the same as responses in ninth grade even for the same students! Of course, the use of eighth graders would be preferred to a sample of sixth graders, but ideally the pilot should occur with ninth graders if the operational form of the survey is intended for ninth graders.

CHAPTER 7

1. **Nominal:** Proportions and frequency distributions could be used.

   Ordinal: Median and/or mode could be used for central tendency. Range could be used for variability. Any of the statistics for nominal-level variables also apply to ordinal-level variables.

Interval: Mean, median, and/or mode could be used for central tendency. Range, standard deviation, and/or variance could be used for variability. Any of the statistics for nominal- or ordinal-level variables also apply to interval-level variables.

Ratio: Mean, median, and/or mode could be used for central tendency. Range, standard deviation, and/or variance could be used for variability. Any of the statistics for nominal-, ordinal-, or interval-level variables also apply to ratio-level variables.

2. Variables measured at the ordinal, interval, or ratio levels can be recoded and treated as the level(s) below it. Lower levels of measurement cannot be moved up the order. Suppose, for example, that an employer conducts an evaluation of its managers, and a score of 10 or higher on this hypothetical survey indicates that employees view the manager(s) favorably. On one hand, if the employer simply collects data on whether or not employees favor their managers, this nominal data can only be summarized with a proportion of employees who favor managers. On the other hand, if the employer records the raw scores (i.e., interval-level variable) of the employees, the data can be used to compute the mean score of its employees as well as the standard deviation. The employer could also recode the data into the "Favorable" or "Unfavorable" category after the fact. Again, data collected at higher metric levels can be treated at its level or any metric level below it.

3. The items with the highest mean scores were Items 10 and 11 (mean = 3.12).

4. The item with the most variability was Item 14 (SD = 1.123).

5. The two items with the strongest correlation were items 6 and 7 (r = .112). This correlation is not very strong, but it is the strongest (i.e., farthest from zero) of those in the correlation table.

6. The two items with the weakest correlation were Items 5 and 9 (r = .032). This correlation was the closest to zero of those in the correlation table.

CHAPTER 8

1. The most frequently chosen response option was "Agree" (n = 109; 36.5%). Slightly more than one-third of the students selected "Agree" to this item, which is acceptable from a measurement perspective. (We are certain the teachers wished 100% of students "Agreed" or "Strongly agreed" with that item!) In order to perform statistical analysis on a set of item responses, the responses must contain variability. That is, respondents use each of the response options provided. Respondents tend not to use all response options for items that are very extremely worded and/or are polarizing. The distribution of response frequencies indicates that the item quality is acceptable from a measurement perspective.

2. The item–total correlation for this item was 0.34, which exceeds the lower acceptable bound of 0.20.

3. The maximum possible score for the item was 4, so the mean of 3.5 is very near the maximum. The mean tells the researcher that the scores are very high, on average, and there is likely very little variability. Although it is a great finding that student report having friends at school, from a measurement perspective

the item does not contribute very much information (i.e., variability) about students. Therefore, its quality is limited.

4. From a statistical perspective, yes, we would absolutely include the item. The major consideration is whether or not the item reflects student engagement as the scale is intended to measure. This determination will in large part be based on the conceptual framework that was developed prior to the development of items (see Chapter 3). An argument could be made for including the item in a student engagement scale because students who feel that their teachers care about them are more likely to be engaged; so the item is related to student engagement. If this item were theoretically justified for inclusion, the item–total correlation definitely supports its inclusion because the correlation is strong.

5. The literature review contributes primarily to the evidence collected to support content validity, which is an important component for construct validity. The literature helps the researchers establish the boundaries of the construct being studied. As a result, the items developed to measure the construct are more likely to represent the construct because it is well defined.

6. The correlation between the two related measures of job satisfaction provides evidence for the instrument's criterion-related validity. In such a case, the supervisors' overall job satisfaction ratings are the criterion against which the survey results are compared.

7. A reliability coefficient of 0.85 is acceptable for nearly any measurement purpose, including measuring job satisfaction. The lower bound of acceptable reliability is often determined by use of the data collected with an instrument. When high-stakes decisions are made based on survey results, reliability coefficients of 0.85 or higher are desired. In the context of measuring job satisfaction, a reliability coefficient of 0.70 may even be acceptable. Again, a reliability coefficient of 0.85 is acceptable.

CHAPTER 9

1. No. The first bit of output to consider is in the Total Variance Explained table in the column labeled "Extraction Sums of Squared Loadings." The Kaiser criterion of eigenvalues greater than 1.0 can be applied to this column. The first extracted factor has an eigenvalue of 7.625, and the second extracted factor has an eigenvalue of 0.517. This supports the extraction of only one factor. Next, we consider the scree plot. The plot appears to level off (i.e., elbow) at the second extracted factor. This supports the extraction of only one factor. We also consider the Pattern Matrix table. Using a minimum cutoff of 0.4, Items 1 through 10 load onto Factor 1, and only Items 11 and 12 load onto Factor 2. This suggests that Factor 2 may not be adequately covered by the items, and the majority of the items load together on Factor 1. Next, we consider the Factor Correlation Matrix table. The estimated correlation between Factors 1 and 2 is 0.802, which is very high. The correlation is so high, in fact, that one may consider them to be the same factor. Taken together, the output from the exploratory factor analysis does not support the researcher's conceptualization of a two-factor solution. The output supports a single-factor solution.

2. The review of the Index of Teaching Stress (ITS) includes only brief mention of factor analysis specifically. One might reasonably expect from the "Scores" section at the beginning of the review that many factors would be extracted from the data because there are multiple scores in addition to the Total Teacher Stress score. In the "DESCRIPTION" section of the actual review, the reviewer states that there are 90 items divided into three domains. The first domain (i.e., Attention-Deficit/Hyperactivity) is measured by 16 items; the second domain (i.e., Student Characteristics) includes four subscales measured by a total of 31 items; and the third domain (i.e., Teacher Characteristics) includes four subscales measured by a total of 43 items. Yet, in the "DEVELOPMENT" section of the review, the reviewer reports that factor analysis of the 90 items yielded two factors. She goes on to report that the ITS developers do provide reasoning for why a third factor was added. In order to fully evaluate the quality of the psychometric properties of the instrument, additional information would be beneficial. The provided review, though generally positive, leaves one to wonder about the statistical justification for so many scores (i.e., at least nine) being produced by an instrument for which factor analysis identified two factors.

CHAPTER 10

1. Here is a revised version of the table. Notice that the percentages are arranged from high to low.

Frequency of Reported Classroom Assessment Practices Used to Monitor Student Progress	
Assessment practice	Frequency (percentage)
Writing samples	97.9
Conferencing with students	92.7
Kidwatching/observation	88.4
Anecdotal notes	70.2
Spelling tests	67.7
Teacher-made tests (e.g., multiple choice, short answer, matching)	65.8
Student portfolios	65.3
Running records	65.0
Core reading tests (supplied by publisher)	60.3
Vocabulary tests	52.6
Miscue analysis	41.8

2. The figure more readily allows the reader to compare the means of the respondents classified as "Pass" or "Fail" because the height of the bars can be directly compared due to their proximity. The table makes comparing the means much more difficult. It is much easier to see that the Pass group has higher mean

responses for the first five items and lower mean responses for the sixth item. Revised versions of the table and bar graphs are below.

Student Ratings on the Student/Teacher Interaction Scale by Pass and Fail for Mathematics

	Test result						Mean difference[a]
	Pass			Fail			
Statement	N	Mean	SD	N	Mean	SD	
My math teacher calls students by their names.	208	3.65	0.65	87	3.55	0.73	0.10
My math teacher tries to be helpful.	202	3.32	0.84	87	2.87	0.99	0.45
My math teacher compliments student successes.	208	3.00	0.95	87	2.64	1.00	0.36
My math teacher cares about what students have to say.	206	2.99	0.90	86	2.53	0.94	0.46
My math teacher has a sense of humor.	209	2.69	0.96	86	2.28	1.08	0.41
My math teacher puts students down for mistakes.	209	1.54	0.81	87	1.85	0.92	−0.31

[a]Positive mean difference indicates that the mean of the Pass group was higher than that of the Fail group. Negative mean difference indicates that the mean of the Fail group was higher than that of the Pass group.

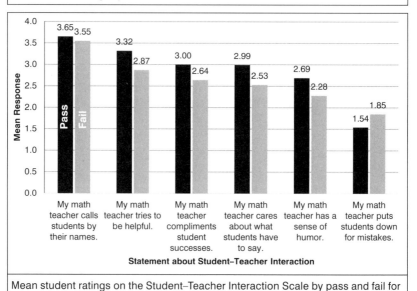

Mean student ratings on the Student–Teacher Interaction Scale by pass and fail for mathematics.

3. We would definitely use the Introduction to acquaint the reader with the background and purpose served by the instrument. Highlight should also be

considered in this case. For example, the mean responses were higher for the Pass group than for the Fail group on five of the six items. For several of the items, the difference was nearly half a scale point, which may be a substantively important call to the reader's attention. Because of the content included in the sixth item, Inquiring narrative may also be considered. Administrators may be interested to know if teachers are putting students down for making mistakes regardless of the students' testing outcomes. The type(s) of narrative selected to accompany tables and figures may be impacted by the context and/or purpose of the instrument.

APPENDIX

1. The primary difference between descriptive and inferential statistics is related to the type of conclusions the researcher is attempting to reach. Descriptive statistics are used to describe the characteristics (e.g., central tendency, variability) of a sample. They are also used as point estimates of population parameters. Inferential statistics are used to make inferences about the characteristics of a population based on the information provided by samples. When using descriptive statistics to describe a sample, the researcher is not making any effort to apply the information from the sample beyond the sample. That is, she is not trying to make an inference about a population parameter. In order to make an inference with some degree of confidence, the researcher must often make assumptions about the distributions. The accuracy of one's inferences is related to the tenability of the distributional assumptions.

2. Responses to this question are likely to vary. Generally, descriptive statistics may be preferable to inferential analysis if *only* one type of analysis were possible. As mentioned previously, descriptive analysis is used to describe the sample with certainty. Descriptive can also be used to estimate a population parameter, but the estimate is not associated with any confidence. To apply confidence to the estimate, inferential analysis is needed, but its accuracy is based on the tenability of distributional assumptions.

3. **One-sample *t*-test**: The board of directors at a local hospital system is considering launching a new advertising campaign depending on its level of patient satisfaction. A researcher working with the board recommends a patient satisfaction survey that was normed with a nationally representative sample of patients. The mean satisfaction rating in the national sample was 15 out of 30. With the approval of the hospital's institution review board, the researcher administers the survey to a random sample of patients for whom the hospital provided services within the past 5 years. In order to determine whether the hospital's patients have higher mean satisfaction than the national average, the researcher could conduct a one-sample *t*-test.

Dependent-samples *t*-test: The board of directors at a local hospital decides to implement a new employee assistance program for its nursing staff. In order to determine if the employee assistance program has an impact on the nursing staff's satisfaction, they administered a satisfaction survey before implementing the employee assistance program and several months afterward. A dependent-samples *t*-test could be used to determine whether there was improvement in the mean satisfaction scores of the nursing staff.

Independent-samples *t*-test: A dentist recently purchased a machine to make crowns in-house rather than sending a model of the patients' teeth to a local dental lab. She is interested in determining whether patients have different satisfaction levels depending on whether the crown was made in-house versus sent off to the dental lab. With the approval of an institutional review board on the research protocol, the dentist randomly determines if patients within a two-month period have their crowns made in-house or in the dental lab. Three months later, the dentist administers a survey to the patients to determine their satisfaction with their crowns. An independent-samples *t*-test could be used to compare the mean satisfaction scores between the two sets of patients.

Analysis of variance: A local doctor is interested in the reported pain level of recovering patients who underwent hernia repair surgery using one of three surgical techniques: open, laparoscopic, or robotic-assisted. With the approval of the hospital's institution review board, the doctor administers a survey to measure the pain levels experienced by patients during recovery. To determine if the mean pain levels were the same or different across surgical techniques, one-way ANOVA could be used on the reported pain scores.

References

Abidin, R. (1983). *Parenting Stress Index*. Charlottesville, VA: Pediatric Psychology Press.

Abidin, R. (1995). *Parenting Stress Index: Professional manual* (3rd ed.). Odessa, FL: Psychological Assessment Resources.

Abidin, R., Greene, R., & Konold, T. (2003). *Index of teaching stress*. Lutz, FL: Psychological Assessment Resources.

Agresti, A., & Finlay, B. (2008). *Statistical methods for the social sciences* (4th ed.). Upper Saddle River, NJ: Prentice Hall.

Allen, E., & Seaman, J. (2006). Making the grade: Online education in the United States, 2006. Retrieved January 14, 2013, from *http://sloanconsortium.org/ publications/freedownloads*.

American Educational Research Association (AERA). (2013). 2013 annual meeting call for submissions. Retrieved from *www.aera.net*.

American Educational Research Association (AERA), American Psychological Association (APA), & National Council on Measurement in Education (NCME). (2014). *Standards for educational and psychological testing*. Washington, DC: AERA.

American Psychological Association. (2010). *Publication manual of the American Psychological Association* (6th ed.). Washington, DC: Author.

American Psychological Association. (2014). Permissions alert form for APA journal authors. Retrieved from *www.apa.org/pubs/authors/permissions-alert. pdf*.

Andrews, F. M. (1984). Construct validity and error components of survey measures: A structural modeling approach. *Public Opinion Quarterly, 48*(2), 409–442.

Baker, J. (2013). Walking the copyright tightrope. *AORN Journal, 97*(2), 167–171.

Bandalos, D., & Enders, C. (1996). The effects of nonnormality and number of response categories on reliability. *Applied Measurement in Education, 9*(2), 151–160.

Barnette, J. (2010). Likert scaling. In N. Salkind (Ed.), *Encyclopedia of research design* (pp. 715–719). Thousand Oaks, CA: Sage.

Becker, W. M. (1976). Biasing effect of respondents' identification on responses to a social desirability scale: A warning to researchers. *Psychological Reports, 39*(3), 756–758.

Bendig, A. (1953). The reliability of self ratings as a function of the amount of verbal anchoring and the number of categories on the scale. *Journal of Applied Psychology, 37*(1), 38–41.

Bendig, A. (1954). Reliability and the number of rating scale categories. *Journal of Applied Psychology, 38*(1), 38–40.

Ben-Shakhar, G., & Sinai, Y. (1991). Gender differences in multiple-choice tests: The role of differential guessing tendencies. *Journal of Educational Measurement, 28*, 23–35.

Betts, L., & Hartley, J. (2012). The effects of changes in the order of verbal labels and numerical values on children's scores on attitude and rating scales. *British Educational Research Journal, 38*(2), 319–331.

Bevan, M., Denton, J., & Myers, J. (1974). The robustness of the *F* test to violations of continuity and form of treatment population. *British Journal of Mathematical and Statistical Psychology, 27*(2), 199–204.

Bishop, G., Tuchfarber, A., & Oldendick, R. (1986). Opinions on fictitious issues: The pressure to answer survey questions. *Public Opinion Quarterly, 50*, 240–250.

Box, G. (1953). Non-normality and tests on variance. *Biometrika, 40*, 318–335.

Box, G. (1954). Some theorems on quadratic forms applied in the study of analysis of variance problems: I. Effect of inequality of variance in the one-way classification. *Annals of Mathematical Statistics, 25*, 290–302.

Brown, T. (2006). *Confirmatory factor analysis for applied research.* New York: Guilford Press.

Brown, T. A. (2015). *Confirmatory factor analysis for applied research* (2nd ed.). New York: Guilford Press.

Buja, A., & Eyuboglu, N. (1992). Remarks on parallel analysis. *Multivariate Behavioral Research, 27*, 509–540.

Camilli, G. (2006). Test fairness. In R. Brennan (Ed.), *Educational measurement* (4th ed., pp. 221–256). Westport, CT: American Council on Education and Praeger.

Cattell, R. B. (1966). The scree test for the number of factors. *Multivariate Behavioral Research, 1*(2), 245–276.

Chow, S. (2010). Research hypothesis. In N. Salkind (Ed.), *Encyclopedia of research design* (pp. 1260–1261). Thousand Oaks, CA: Sage.

Clauser B., & Mazor, K. (1998). Using statistical procedures to identify differentially functioning test items. *Educational Measurement: Issues and Practice, 17*(1), 281–294.

Cochran, W. G. (1977). *Sampling techniques* (3rd ed.). New York: Wiley.

Cohen, J. (1977). *Statistical power analysis for the behavioral sciences.* Hillsdale, NJ: Erlbaum.

Cohen, J. (1988). *Statistical power analysis for the behavioral sciences* (2nd ed.). Hillsdale, NJ: Erlbaum.

Colton, D., & Covert, R. (2007). *Designing and constructing instruments for social research and evaluation*. San Francisco: Jossey-Bass.

Comrey, A. L., & Lee, H. B. (1992). *A first course in factor analysis*. Hillsdale, NJ: Erlbaum.

Conover, W. (1999). *Practical nonparametric statistics*. New York: Wiley.

Copyright Clearance Center. (2013). Top ten misconceptions about copyright. Retrieved from *Copyright.com*.

Cortina, J. M. (1993). What is coefficient alpha?: An examination of theory and applications. *Journal of Applied Psychology, 78*(1), 98–104.

Couper, M., Traugott, M., & Lamias, M. (2001). Web survey design and administration. *Public Opinion Quarterly, 65*(2), 230–253.

Crespi, I. (1971). What kinds of attitude measures are predictive of behavior? *Public Opinion Quarterly, 35,* 327–334.

Crocker, A., & Algina, J. (2006). *Introduction to classical and modern test theory*. New York: Holt, Rinehart & Winston.

Crocker, L. (2001). Content validity. In N. Smelser & P. Baltes (Eds.), *International encyclopedia of the social and behavioral sciences* (pp. 2702–2705). Kidlington, Oxford, UK: Elsevier.

Cronbach, L. (1946). Response sets and test validity. *Educational and Psychological Measurement, 6,* 475–494.

Cronbach, L. (1950). Further evidence on response sets and test design. *Educational and Psychological Measurement, 10,* 3–31.

Davis, F. B. (1964). *Educational measurements and their interpretation*. Belmont CA: Wadsworth.

Dawes, J. (2008). Do data characteristics change according to the number of scale points used?: An experiment using 5-point, 7-point and 10-point scales. *International Journal of Market Research, 50*(1), 61–77.

De Ayala, R. J. (2009). *The theory and practice of item response theory*. New York: Guilford Press.

DeVellis, R. (2012). *Scale development: Theory and applications* (3rd ed.). Thousand Oaks, CA: Sage.

Dillman, D., Smyth, J., & Christian, L. (2009). *Internet, mail, and mixed-mode surveys: The tailored design method* (3rd ed.). Hoboken, NJ: Wiley.

DiPerna, J., & Elliott, S. (1999). Development and validation of the Academic Competence Evaluation Scales. *Journal of Psychoeducational Assessment, 17,* 207–225.

DiPerna, J., & Elliott, S. (2000). *Academic Competence Evaluation Scales*. San Antonio, TX: Pearson.

DiStefano, C., Zhu, M., & Mîndrilă, D. (2009). Understanding and using factor scores: Considerations for the applied researcher. *Practical Assessment, Research and Evaluation, 14*(20), 1–11. Available at *http://pareonline.net/getvn.asp?v=14&n=20.*

Duhachek, A., & Iacobucci, D. (2004). Alpha's standard error (ASE): An accurate and precise confidence interval estimate. *Journal of Applied Psychology, 89*(5), 792–808.

Earp, J., & Ennett, S. (1991). Conceptual models for health education research and practice. *Health Education Research: Theory and Practice, 6*(2), 163–171.

Ebel, R. (1965). *Measuring educational achievement* (2nd ed.). Englewood Cliffs, NJ: Prentice Hall.

Educational Testing Service. (2014). The *Test Collection at ETS*: Index of Teaching Stress. Retrieved from *www.ets.org/test_link/about.*

Ehrenberg, A. (1977). Rudiments of numeracy. *Journal of the Royal Statistical Society, Series A, 140,* 277–297.

Enders, C., & Bandalos, D. (1999). The effects of heterogeneous item distributions on reliability. *Applied Measurement in Education, 9*(2), 151–160.

Evergreen, S. (2014). *Presenting data effectively: Communicating your findings for maximum impact.* Thousand Oaks, CA: Sage.

Everitt, B., & Skrondal, A. (2010). *The Cambridge dictionary of statistics* (4th ed.). Cambridge, UK: Cambridge University Press.

Fabrigar, L., Wegener, D., MacCallum, R., & Strahan, E. (1999). Evaluating the use of exploratory factor analysis in psychological research. *Psychological Methods, 4*(3), 272–299.

Fabrigar, L., & Wood, J. (2007). Likert scaling. In N. Salkind (Ed.), *Encyclopedia of measurement and statistics* (Vol. 1, pp. 536–540). Thousand Oaks, CA: Sage.

Farquhar, A., & Farquhar, H. (1891). *Economic and industrial delusions: A discourse of the case for protection.* New York: Putnam.

Fawcett, J. (1995). *Analysis and evaluation of conceptual models of nursing* (3rd ed.). Philadelphia: Davis.

Fazio, R., & Olson, M. (2007). Attitudes: Foundations, functions, and consequences. In M. Hogg & J. Cooper (Eds.), *The Sage handbook of social psychology: Concise student edition* (pp. 123–146). Thousand Oaks, CA: Sage.

Few, S. (2004). *Show me the numbers.* Oakland, CA: Analytics Press.

Fink, A. (1995). *How to ask survey questions.* Thousand Oaks, CA: Sage.

Fink, A. (2002). *How to report on surveys* (2nd ed.). Thousand Oaks, CA: Sage.

Fink, A. (2003). *How to ask survey questions* (2nd ed.). Thousand Oaks, CA: Sage.

Fink, A. (2013). *How to conduct surveys: A step-by-step guide* (5th ed.). Thousand Oaks, CA: Sage.

Fishman, S. (2011). *The copyright handbook: What every writer needs to know* (11th ed.). Berkeley, CA: Nolo.

Fowler, F. (1995). *Improving survey questions: Design and evaluation.* Thousand Oaks, CA: Sage.

Fowler, F. (2014). *Survey research methods* (5th ed.). Thousand Oaks, CA: Sage.

Fraenkel, J., & Wallen, N. (2009). *How to design and evaluate research in education* (7th ed.). Boston: McGraw-Hill.

Francis, J., & Busch, L. (1975). What we now know about "I don't knows." *Public Opinion Quarterly, 39*(2), 207–218.

Frary, R. (2003). A brief guide to questionnaire development. Retrieved from *www.peecworks.org/PEEC/PEEC_Inst/I0004E536.*

Furr, R., & Bacharach, V. (2009). *Psychometrics: An introduction.* Thousand Oaks, CA: Sage.

Gall, M., Gall, J., & Borg, W. (2010). *Applying educational research: How to read, do, and use research to solve problems of practice* (7th ed.). Boston: Pearson.

Gambrell, L., Palmer, B., Codling, R., & Mazzoni, S. (1996). Assessing motivation to read. *The Reading Teacher,* 518–533.

Geisinger, K., Spies, R., Carlson, J., & Plake, B. (Eds.). (2007). *The seventeenth mental measurements yearbook*. Lincoln, NE: Buros Institute of Mental Measurement.

Glatthorn, A. (1998). *Writing the winning dissertation: A step-by-step guide*. Thousand Oaks, CA: Sage.

Goddard III, R., & Villanova, P. (2006). Designing surveys and questionnaires for research. In F. Leong & J. Austin (Eds.), *The psychology research handbook: A guide for graduate students and research assistants* (2nd ed., pp. 114–124). Thousand Oaks, CA: Sage.

Gorsuch, R. (1983). *Factor analysis* (2nd ed.). Hillsdale, NJ: Erlbaum.

Greca, I., & Moreira, M. (2000). Mental models, conceptual models, and modeling. *International Journal of Science Education, 22*(1), 1–11.

Green, P., & Rao, V. (1970). Rating scales and information recovery—How many scales and response categories to use. *Journal of Marketing, 34*(3), 33–39.

Guilford Press. (2014). Permission request form. Retrieved from *www.guilford.com/authors*.

Gustav, A. (1963). Response sets in objective achievement tests. *Journal of Psychology, 56*, 421–427.

Hao, S., & Johnson, R. (2013). Teachers' classroom assessment practices and fourth graders' reading literacy achievements: An international study. *Teaching and Teacher Education, 29*, 53–63.

Harman, H. (1976). *Modern factor analysis* (3rd ed.). Chicago: University of Chicago Press.

Hartley, J., & Betts, L. (2010). Four layouts and a finding: The effects of changes in the order of the verbal labels and numerical values on Likert-type scales. *International Journal of Social Research Methodology, 13*(1), 17–27.

Hatcher, L. (1994). *Step-by-step approach to using the SAS system for factor analysis and structural equation modeling*. Cary, NC: SAS Institute.

Heeren, T., & Agostino, R. (1987). Robustness of the two independent samples *t*-test when applied to ordinal scaled data. *Statistics in Medicine, 6*, 79–90.

Helm, E., Sedlacek, W., & Prieto, D. (1998). The relationship between attitudes toward diversity and overall satisfaction of university students by race. *Journal of College Counseling, 1*(2), 111–120.

Herman, J., Aschbacher, P., & Winters, L. (1992). *A practical guide to alternative assessment*. Alexandria, VA: Association for Supervision and Curriculum Development.

Hill, R. (2002, April). *Examining the reliability of accountability systems*. Paper presented at the annual meeting of the American Educational Research Association, New Orleans, LA.

Holbrook, A. (2008). Acquiescence response bias. In P. Lavrakas (Ed.), *Encyclopedia of survey research methods* (pp. 3–4). Thousand Oaks, CA: Sage.

Hopkins, K. (1998). *Educational and psychological measurement and evaluation* (8th ed.). Englewood Cliffs, NJ: Prentice Hall.

Hough, H., & Priddy, K. (2012). Copyright and the perioperative nurse. *Perioperative Nursing Clinics, 7*(2), 201–210.

Hsu, T., & Feldt, L. (1969). The effect of limitations on the number of criterion score values on the significance level of the *F*-test. *American Educational Research Journal, 6*(4), 515–527.

Hubbard, R., & McIntosh, J. (1992). Integrating suicidology into abnormal psychology classes: The Revised Facts on Suicide Quiz. *Teaching of Psychology, 3,* 163–165.

Humphreys, L. G., & Montanelli, R. G. (1975). An investigation of the parallel analysis criterion for determining the number of common factors. *Multivariate Behavioral Research, 10*(2), 193–205.

Jaeger, R. M. (1984). *Sampling in education and the social sciences.* New York: Longman.

Johnson, R. L. (1996). *Family educators' responses to the portfolio assessment review.* Lincoln, NE: Educational Service Unit Number 18.

Johnson, R. L., Davis, K., Fisher, S., Johnson, C., & Somerindyke, J. (2000). *Evaluation of the Transition Program of Richland School District Two.* Columbia: College of Education, University of South Carolina.

Johnson, R. L., Davis, K., Fisher, S., & Somerindyke, J. (2001, November). *Variability in student ratings of instructional practices in English and mathematics classes: Implications for instrument development.* Paper presented at the annual meeting of the American Evaluation Association, St. Louis, MO.

Johnson, R. L., Green, S., Kim, D., & Pope, N. (2008). Educational leaders' perceptions about ethical assessment practices. *American Journal of Evaluation, 29*(4), 520–530.

Johnson, R. L., Monrad, D., Amsterdam, C., & May, J. (2005). *An evaluation of the High School Initiatives 2000+ of Richland School District Two.* Columbia: University of South Carolina.

Kaiser, H. F. (1960). The application of electronic computers to factor analysis. *Educational and Psychological Measurement, 20,* 141–151.

Kane, M. (1982). A sampling model for validity. *Applied Psychological Measurement, 6*(2), 125–160.

Kane, M. (2001). Current concerns in validity theory. *Journal of Educational Measurement, 38*(4), 319–342.

Kane, M. (2009). Validating the interpretations and uses of test scores. In R. Lissitz (Ed.), *The concept of validity: Revisions, new directions, and applications* (pp. 39–64). Charlotte, NC: Information Age.

Kaplan, R., & Saccuzzo, D. (1982). *Psychological testing: Principles, applications, and issues.* Monterey, CA: Brooks/Cole.

Kear, D., Coffman, G., McKenna, M., & Ambrosio, A. (2000). Measuring attitude toward writing: A new tool for teachers. *The Reading Teacher, 54*(1), 10–23.

Kirk, R. E. (2008). *Statistics: An introduction* (5th ed.). Belmont, CA: Thomson.

Kline, R. B. (2015). *Principles and practice of structural equation modeling* (4th ed.). New York: Guilford Press.

Kouzes, J., & Posner, B. (2002). *Leadership Practices Inventory (LPI)* (3rd ed.). San Francisco: Jossey-Bass.

Krebs, D., & Hoffmeyer-Zlotnik, J. (2010). Positive first or negative first?: Effects of the order of answering categories on response behavior. *Methodology, 6*(3), 118–127.

Krosnick, J., & Fabrigar, L. (1997). Designing rating scales for effective measurement in surveys. In L. Lyberg, P. Biemer, M. Collins, E. de Leeuw, C. Dippo, N. Schwarz, et al. (Eds.), *Survey measurement and process quality* (pp. 141–164). Hoboken, NJ: Wiley.

Kyriakidou, O. (2009). Attitude and attitude change. In C. Wankel (Ed.), *Encyclopedia of business in today's world* (pp. 87–90). Thousand Oaks, CA: Sage.

Leeuw, E., Hox, J., & Dillman, D. (2008). The cornerstone of survey research. In E. Leeuw, J. Hox, & D. Dillman (Eds.), *International handbook of survey methodology* (pp. 1–34). New York: Psychology Press.

Levene, H. (1960). Robust tests for equality of variances. In I. Olkin, S. Ghurye, W. Hoeffding, W. Madow, & H. Mann (Eds.), *Contributions to probability and statistics: Essays in honor of Harold Hotelling* (pp. 278–292). Palo Alto, CA: Stanford University Press.

Lord, F. M. (1953). On the statistical treatment of football numbers. *American Psychologist, 8*(12), 750–751.

Lozano, L., García-Cueto, E., & Muñiz, J. (2008). Effect of the number of response categories on the reliability and validity of rating scales. *Methodology, 4*(2), 73–79.

Lunney, G. H. (1970). Using analysis of variance with a dichotomous outcome variable. *Journal of Educational Measurement, 7*(4), 263–269.

MacCallum, R., Widaman, K., Preacher, K., & Hong, S. (2001). Sample size in factor analysis: The role of model error. *Multivariate Behavioral Research, 36*, 611–637.

MacCallum, R., Widaman, K., Zhang, S., & Hong, S. (1999). Sample size in factor analysis. *Psychological Methods, 4*, 84–99.

Macmillan-McGraw Hill. (1993). *Reflecting diversity: Multicultural guidelines for educational publishing professionals.* New York: Author.

Maitland, A. (2009). Should I label all scale points of just the end points for attitudinal questions? Retrieved from *http://surveypractice.org.*

Marascuilo, L., & McSweeney, M. (1977). *Nonparametric and distribution-free methods for the social sciences.* Monterey, CA: Brooks/Cole.

Margoluis, R., & Salafsky, N. (1998). *Measures of success: Designing, managing, and monitoring conservation and development projects.* Washington, DC: Island Press.

Masters, J. (1974). The relationship between number of response categories and reliability of Likert-type questionnaires. *Journal of Educational Measurement, 11*(1), 49–53.

Matwin, S., & Fabrigar, L. (2007). Attitude tests. In N. Salkind (Ed.), *Encyclopedia of measurement and statistics* (Vol. 1, pp. 53–56). Thousand Oaks, CA: Sage.

Maxwell, J. (2013). *Qualitative research design: An interactive approach* (3rd ed.). Thousand Oaks, CA: Sage.

Mazaheri, M., & Theuns, P. (2009). Effects of varying response formats on self-ratings of life-satisfaction. *Social Indicators Research, 90*(3), 381–395.

McDavid, J., & Hawthorn, L. (2006). *Program evaluation and performance measurement: An introduction to practice.* Thousand Oaks, CA: Sage.

McKenna, M., & Kear, D. (1999). Measuring attitude toward reading: A new tool for teachers. In S. Barrentine (Ed.), *Reading assessment: Principles and practices for elementary teachers* (pp. 199–214). Newark, DE: International Reading Association.

Mertler, C., & Vannatta, R. (2005). *Advanced and multivariate statistical analysis.* Los Angeles: Pyrczak.

Messick, S. (1991). Psychology and methodology of response styles. In R. Snow & D. Wiley (Eds.), *Improving inquiry in social science* (pp. 161–200). Hillsdale, NJ: Erlbaum.

Messick, S. (1993). Validity. In R. Linn (Ed.), *Educational measurement* (3rd ed., pp. 13–103). Washington, DC: American Council on Education.

Meyer, J. P. (2010). *Reliability.* New York: Oxford University Press.

Meyer, J. P., & Seaman, M. A. (2008). A comparison of the exact Kruskal–Wallis distribution to asymptotic approximations for all sample sizes up to 105. *Journal of Experimental Education, 81*(2), 139–156.

Microsoft Corporation. (2010). *Test your document's readability.* Redmond, WA: Author.

Miles, M., & Huberman, A. (1994). *Qualitative data analysis: An expanded sourcebook.* Thousand Oaks, CA: Sage.

Monrad, D., May, R. J., DiStefano, C., Smith, J., Gay, J., Mîndrilă, D., et al. (2008, March). *Parent, student, and teacher perceptions of school climate: Investigations across organizational levels.* Paper presented at the annual meeting of the American Educational Research Association, New York.

Montei, M., Adams, G., & Eggers, L. (1996). Validity of scores on the attitudes toward diversity scale (ATDS). *Educational and Psychological Measurement, 56*(2), 293–303.

Morgan, G., Sherlock, J., & Ritchie, W. (2010). Job satisfaction in the home health care context: Validating a customized instrument for application. *Journal of Healthcare Management, 55*(1), 11–23.

Murray-Ward, M. (2007). [Review of the *Index of Teaching Stress*, by R. Abidin, R. Greene, & T. Konold, 2003]. *Mental Measurements Yearbook, 17.* Retrieved from *http://buros.org.*

Nanna, M., & Sawilowsky, S. (1998). Analysis of Likert scale data in disability and medical rehabilitation research. *Psychological Methods, 3*(1), 55–67.

Nardi, P. (2003). *Doing survey research: A guide to quantitative methods.* Boston: Pearson Education.

Nathan, G. (2008). Internet surveys. In P. Lavrakas (Ed.), *Encyclopedia of survey research methods* (pp. 356–359). Thousand Oaks, CA: Sage.

Nicholls, M., Orr, C., Okubo, M., & Loftus, A. (2006). Satisfaction guaranteed: The effect of spatial biases on responses to Likert scales. *Psychological Science, 17*(12), 1027–1028.

Nitko, A. (n.d.). *Using a Mental Measurements Yearbook review and other materials to evaluate a test.* Lincoln, NE: Buros Center for Testing. Retrieved from *http://buros.org/educational-resources.*

Nitko, A. (2014). *Using a Mental Measurements Yearbook review to evaluate a test.* Lincoln, NE: Buros Center for Testing. Retrieved from *http://buros.org.*

Nunnally, J. (1978). *Psychometric theory* (2nd ed.). New York: McGraw-Hill.

Office of Program Evaluation/South Carolina Educational Policy Center. (2005). *South Carolina Reading First Initiative: Classroom teacher survey instrument.* Columbia: College of Education, University of South Carolina.

Oppenheim, A. (1992). *Questionnaire design, interviewing and attitude measurement.* London: Pinter.

Orcher, L. (2007). *Conducting a survey: Techniques for a term project.* Glendale, CA: Pyrczak.

Ostrom, T. (1971). Item construction in attitude measurement. *Public Opinion Quarterly, 35*(4), 593–600.

Paulhus, D. (1991). Measurement and control of response bias. In J. Robinson, P. Shaver, & L. Wrightsman (Eds.), *Measures of personality and social psychological attitudes* (pp. 17–59). San Diego, CA: Academic Press.

Pearson, P. D. (2004). The reading wars. *Educational Policy, 18*(1), 216–252.

Pedhazur, E. J., & Schmelkin, L. P. (1991). *Measurement, design, and analysis: An integrated approach.* Hillsdale, NJ: Erlbaum.

Peer, E., & Gamliel, E. (2011). Too reliable to be true?: Response bias as a potential source of inflation in paper-and-pencil questionnaire reliability. *Practical Assessment, Research and Evaluation, 16*(9), 1–8.

Penman, A., & Johnson, W. (2006). The changing shape of the body mass index distribution curve in the population: Implications for public health policy to reduce the prevalence of adult obesity. *Preventing Chronic Disease, 3*(3), 1–4.

Peterson, R. (1997). A quantitative analysis of rating-scale response variability. *Marketing Letters, 8*(1), 9–21.

Peterson, R. (2000). *Constructing effective questionnaires.* Thousand Oaks, CA: Sage.

Pew Research Center. (2007). Global unease with major world powers: Rising environmental concern in 47-nation survey. Retrieved from *www.pewglobal.org.*

Phillips, S. (2000, April). Legal corner: GI forum v TEA. *NCME Newsletter,* 8.

Presser, S., & Schuman, H. (1980). The measurement of a middle position in attitude surveys. *Public Opinion Quarterly, 44*(1), 70–85.

Ravitch, S., & Riggan, M. (2012). *Reason and rigor: How conceptual frameworks guide research.* Thousand Oaks, CA: Sage.

Raymond, M. R. (2005). An NCME instructional module on developing and administering practice analysis questionnaires. *Educational Measurement: Issues and Practice, 24*(2), 29–42.

Research Committee of the Sierra Club. (n.d.). *Environmental priorities survey.* San Francisco: Author.

Riconscente, M., & Romeo, I. (2010). A technique for the measurement of attitudes. In N. Salkind (Ed.), *Encyclopedia of research design* (pp. 1490–1493). Thousand Oaks, CA: Sage.

Robson, C. (1993). *Real world research: A resource for social scientists and practitioner–researchers.* Cambridge, MA: Blackwell.

Salkind, N. (2012). *Tests and measurement for people who (think they) hate tests and measurement.* Thousand Oaks, CA: Sage.

Sax, G., with Newton, J. (1997). *Principles of educational and psychological measurement and evaluation* (4th ed.). Belmont, CA: Wadsworth.

Scholderer, J. (2011). Attitude surveys. In D. Southerton (Ed.), *Encyclopedia of consumer culture* (pp. 70–71). Thousand Oaks, CA: Sage.

Schuman, H., & Presser, S. (1996). *Questions and answers in attitude surveys: Experiments on question form, wording, and context.* Thousand Oaks, CA: Sage.

Schwarz, N., Knäuper, B., Hippler, H., Noelle-Neumann, E., & Clark, L. (1991). Rating scales numeric values may change the meaning of scale labels. *Public Opinion Quarterly, 55,* 570–582.

Schwarz, N., Knäuper, B., Oyserman, D., & Stich, C. (2008). The psychology of asking questions. In E. Leeuw, J. Hox, & D. Dillman (Eds.), *International handbook of survey methodology* (pp. 18–34). New York: Psychology Press.

Segal, D. (2000). Levels of knowledge about suicide facts and myths among younger and older adults. *Clinical Gerontologist, 22*(2), 71–80.

Sheskin, D. J. (2007). *Handbook of parametric and nonparametric statistical procedures* (4th ed.). Boca Raton, FL: Chapman & Hall/CRC.

Sireci, S. (2009). Packing and unpacking sources of validity evidence: History repeats itself again. In R. Lissitz (Ed.), *The concept of validity: Revisions, new directions, and applications* (pp. 19–37). Charlotte, NC: Information Age.

Smith, T. (1995). Little things matter: A sampler of how differences in questionnaire format can affect survey responses. *Proceedings of the American Statistical Association, Survey Research Methods Section* (pp. 1046–1051). Alexandria, VA.

Solomon, D. (2001). Conducting web-based surveys. *Practical Assessment, Research and Evaluation, 7*(19). Retrieved from *http://PAREonline.net*.

South Carolina Educational Policy Center. (2003). *Proposal to evaluate South Carolina's Reading First program*. Columbia: College of Education, University of South Carolina.

Spector, P. (1992). *Summated rating scale construction: An introduction*. Newbury Park, CA: Sage.

Stallings, W., & Gillmore, G. (1971). A note on "accuracy" and "precision." *Journal of Educational Measurement, 8*, 127–129.

Stanley, S. (n.d.). *Factors influencing the successful inclusion of special education students into regular education*. Portland, OR: University of Portland.

Stevens, J. P. (2009). *Applied multivariate statistics for the social sciences* (5th ed.). New York: Routledge.

Streiner, D. L. (2003). Starting at the beginning: An introduction to coefficient alpha and internal consistency. *Journal of Personality Assessment, 80*(1), 99–103.

Streiner, D. L., & Norman, G. (2008). *Health measurement scales: A practical guide to their development and use* (4th ed.). New York: Oxford University Press.

Sue, V. M., & Ritter, L. A. (2012). *Conducting online surveys*. Thousand Oaks, CA: Sage.

Tabachnick, B., & Fidell, L. (2013). *Using multivariate statistics* (6th ed.). Boston: Pearson.

Taylor, D. (2007). The politics and passion of how Johnny should read. In M. Taylor (Ed.), *Whole language teaching, whole-hearted practice: Looking back, looking forward* (pp. 161–201). New York: Peter Lang.

Thorkildsen, T. (2010). Validity of measurement. In N. Salkind (Ed.), *Encyclopedia of research design* (pp. 1592–1597). Thousand Oaks, CA: Sage.

Thorndike, R., & Thorndike-Christ, T. (2010). *Measurement and evaluation in psychology and education* (8th ed.). Boston: Pearson.

Thurstone, L. (1947). *Multiple-factor analysis*. Chicago: University of Chicago Press.

Tourangeau, R., Couper, M., & Conrad, F. (2004). Spacing, position, and order: Interpretive heuristics for visual features of survey questions. *Public Opinion Quarterly, 68*(3), 368–393.

Tourangeau, R., Couper, M., & Conrad, F. (2007). Color, labels, and interpretive heuristics for response scales. *Public Opinion Quarterly, 71*(1), 91–112.

United States Copyright Office. (2006). Copyright in general. Retrieved from *www.copyright.gov/help/faq/faq-general.html.*

United States Copyright Office. (2012). Copyright basics. Retrieved from *www.copyright.gov/circs/circ01.pdf.*

University of Arkansas for Medical Sciences. (2014). Take the senior nutrition quiz. Retrieved from *www.uamshealth.com/HealthLibrary/Default.aspx?Content TypeId=40&ContentID=SeniorNutritionQuiz2.*

University of Kansas Research and Training Center on Independent Living. (2008). *Guidelines for reporting and writing about people with disabilities* (7th ed.). Lawrence, KS: Author.

University of Rochester Medical Center. (2014). What do you know about breast cancer? Retrieved from *www.urmc.rochester.edu/encyclopedia.*

Van Vaerenbergh, Y., & Thomas, T. (2013). Response styles in survey research: A literature review of antecedents, consequences, and remedies. *International Journal of Public Opinion Research, 25*(2), 195–217.

Velicer, W., DiClemente, C. C., & Corriveau, D. P. (1984). Item format and the structure of the personal orientation inventory. *Applied Psychological Measurement, 8,* 409–419.

Villar, A. (2008). Response bias. In P. Lavrakas (Ed.), *Encyclopedia of survey research methods* (pp. 751–753). Thousand Oaks, CA: Sage.

Wainer, H. (1992). Understanding graphs and tables. *Educational Researcher, 21*(1), 14–23.

Wainer, H. (1997). Improving tabular displays, with NAEP tables as examples and inspirations. *Journal of Educational and Behavioral Statistics, 22*(1), 1–30.

Wainer, H. (2010). 14 conversations about three things. *Journal of Educational and Behavioral Statistics, 35*(1), 5–25.

Welch, B. L. (1951). On the comparison of several mean values. *Biometrika, 38,* 330–336.

Wells, H. G. (1904). *Mankind in the making.* New York: Scribner's.

Weng, L. (2004). Impact of the number of response categories and anchor labels on coefficient alpha and test–retest reliability. *Educational and Psychological Measurement, 64*(6), 956–972.

Widaman, K. (2007). Common factors versus components: Principals and principles, errors and misconceptions. In R. Cudeck & R. MacCallum (Eds.), *Factor analysis at 100: Historical developments and future directions* (pp. 177–203). Mahwah, NJ: Erlbaum.

Wienclaw, R. A. (2009). Surveys in sociology research. *Research Starters Sociology, 1,* 1–5.

Wiersma, W., & Jurs, S. (2009). *Research methods in education: An introduction* (9th ed.). Boston: Allyn & Bacon.

Wikipedia. (2010). Copyright Clearance Center. Retrieved from *http:// en.wikipedia.org/wiki/Copyright_Clearance_Center.*

Wikipedia. (2016). Measure twice and cut once. Retrieved from *https:// en.wiktionary.org/wiki/measure_twice_and_cut_once.*

Williams, C. (1979). The nature and development of conceptual frameworks. In

F. Downs & J. Fleming (Eds.), *Issues in nursing research* (pp. 89–106). New York: Appleton-Century-Crofts.

Winter, J. (2010). Response bias. In N. Salkind (Ed.), *Encyclopedia of research design* (pp. 1272–1274). Thousand Oaks, CA: Sage.

Wood, R. (1976). Inhibiting blind guessing: The effect of instructions. *Journal of Educational Measurement, 13*, 297–307.

Wright, D., Gaskell, G., & O'Muircheartaigh, D. (1994). How much is 'quite a bit'? Mapping between numerical values and vague quantifiers. *Applied Cognitive Psychology, 8*(5), 479–496.

Zwick, W., & Velicer, W. (1986). Factor influencing five rules for determining the number of components to retain. *Psychological Bulletin, 99*, 432–442.

Author Index

Note: *f* following a page number indicates a figure; *t* indicates a table.

Subject Index

Note: *f* following a page number indicates a figure; *t* indicates a table

M

Mann–Whitney *U* test, 216–219,
    217*t*
Mean, 105–106, 124–125, 124*t*
Measurement, levels of, 100–103
Measurement error, 121–122, 121*t*
Median, 105
Mental Measurements Yearbook
    (MMY)
    classifications of, 24
    instrument reviews in, 20–21, 24,
        25*f*
Microsoft Word, reading level
    estimation and, 56
Mode, 104–105
Models, function of, 9
Motivation to Read Profile: The
    Reading Survey, construct
    measured, domains,
    operationalization, 11*t*
Multidimensionality, of construct
    factor structure, 148–149,
    149*f*

N

Narratives
    functions of, 9, 36, 37*f*, 38–39
    writing, 44
Needs assessments, surveys and, 6
Nominal data, 100–101
Nonparametric statistics, 75
Nonresponse error, 121, 121*t*
Null hypothesis, 196–198, 206–209,
    213
Numeric labels, positive integers for,
    80

O

Objectivity, item writing and, 51
One-sample *t*-test, 200, 201*f*, 202–205,
    202*f*, 203*f*, 241
One-way analysis of variance, 212–
    216, 213*f*, 213*t*, 214*f*, 215*f*

Open-response survey items,
    advantages and disadvantages
    of, 1–2, 2*f*, 3*t*, 4
Order effect, 136*t*, 137
Ordinal data, 101–102

P

PAF (principal axis factoring), 149–
    150, 154, 157
Parallel analysis, 153–154, 153*t*
Parameters, 193
Parent involvement, measurement of,
    66
Pearson correlation, 113
Pencil-and-paper questionnaires, 92
Personal background, item writing
    and, 67–68
Phenomenon of interest, 1, 3, 4, 6, 8, 9,
    36, 38, 43, 44, 49, 86, 102, 189
Phrasing
    qualifying, 60
    repetitive, 60, 61*f*
Pilot tests, conducting, 97–98
Plagiarism, 30
Population, in statistics, 193
Portfolio Assessment Review,
    construct measured, domains,
    operationalization, 11*t*
Primacy effect, 136*t*, 137
Principal axis factoring (PAF), 149–
    150, 151*f*, 154, 157
Probability, finding for test statistics,
    203
Professional critiques, reviewing,
    19–20
Program evaluations, surveys and, 6
Propositions, definitions and
    statements of, 39–40

Q

Quality; *see* Scale quality
Quantile–quantile (Q–Q) plots,
    200–201, 202*f*
Questionnaires, 12

About the Authors

Robert L. Johnson, PhD, is Professor in the Department of Educational Studies at the University of South Carolina. His research focuses on the ethics of classroom assessment practices and the scoring of performance assessments in the language arts and the visual and performing arts. He also writes about the teaching of program evaluation and involvement of stakeholders in evaluations. Dr. Johnson's research has been published in such journals as *Applied Measurement in Education, Language Assessment Quarterly, Assessing Writing, Teaching and Teacher Education, Assessment and Evaluation in Higher Education,* and the *American Journal of Evaluation.* He teaches courses related to educational research, assessment, survey methodology, and program evaluation.

Grant B. Morgan, PhD, is Associate Professor in the Department of Educational Psychology at Baylor University. His primary methodological research focuses on latent variable models, classification, and psychometrics. His research has been published in such journals as *Structural Equation Modeling, Computational Statistics and Data Analysis, Psychological Assessment, School Psychology Quarterly, Language Assessment Quarterly,* and *Quality and Quantity.* Dr. Morgan has evaluation experience at the local, state, and federal levels, and has extensive experience developing and using survey scales. He teaches graduate-level courses covering latent variable models, item response theory, psychometric theory, measurement and evaluation, experimental design, and research methods.